200
Medication Errors
and How to Avoid Them

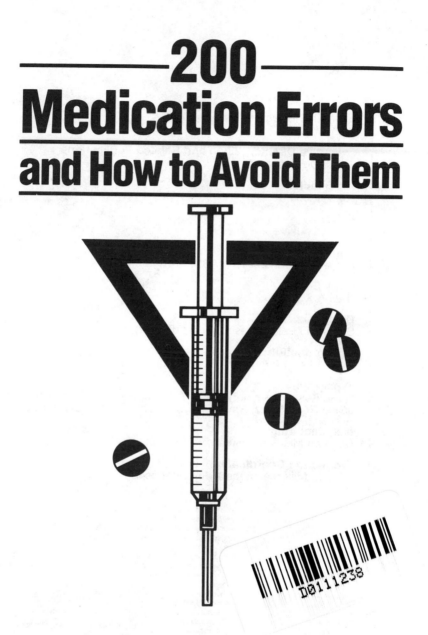

Michael R. Cohen, MS, FASHP

Springhouse Corporation
Springhouse, Pennsylvania

STAFF

Executive Director, Editorial
Stanley Loeb

Executive Director, Video and Related Publications
Jean Robinson

Art Director
John Hubbard

Editor
Susan L. Jackson

Clinical Editor
Michael R. Cohen, MS, FASHP

Copy Editor
Traci A. Ginnona

Designers
Stephanie Peters (associate art director), Kathy Singel

Art Production
Robert Perry (manager), Bob Wieder

Typography
David Kosten (director), Diane Paluba (manager), Elizabeth Bergman, Joyce Rossi Biletz, Phyllis Marron, Robin Rantz, Valerie Rosenberger

Manufacturing
Deborah Meiris (manager), T.A. Landis

Production Coordination
Aline S. Miller (manager), Joy Dickenson

Library of Congress Cataloging-in-Publication Data

Cohen, Michael R. (Michael Richard), 1944–
  200 medication errors and how to avoid
them/by Michael R. Cohen.
    p.   cm.
  Includes index.
  1. Medical errors. I. Title. II. Title: Two hundred medication errors and how to avoid them.
  [DNLM: 1. Medication Errors—nurses' instruction. QZ 42 C678z]
RM146.C64   1991
615.5′8—dc20
DNLM/DLC   90-9832
ISBN 0-87434-311-9   CIP

FOREWORD

Since the first medication error study 20 years ago, dedicated nurses and pharmacists have reported medication errors through our nation's health care systems. These reports indicate that one out of every five doses of medication administered may be given to the wrong patient, in the wrong dose, by the wrong route, at the wrong time, or even as the wrong drug.

In 1975, I began collecting reports of actual medication errors experienced by health care professionals across the country. Nurses and pharmacists have benefited from my sharing of this collection through publication in *Nursing* magazine and *Hospital Pharmacy,* a pharmacy journal for which I serve as assistant editor. Using the model of the airline industry, where accidents are carefully analyzed and preventive recommendations suggested for wide adoption, I hoped this publicity would help health care professionals give safe drug therapy for their patients.

When an error reaches a patient, it's frequently a result of multiple breakdowns in the ordering, dispensing, and administration systems. Rarely is one individual entirely responsible for what has gone wrong. But an informed and aware nurse, at the interface of the drug and the patient, can be the final defense in preventing a medication error from reaching the patient.

All of the errors in this book have happened more than once—perhaps thousands of times. Many have resulted in patient injury or death. All of them have been submitted by concerned readers in the hopes that others could learn from the original errors. I hope the recommendations that go along with each account will be useful in helping you provide safe drug therapy for your patients.

Michael R. Cohen, MS, FASHP
Director of Pharmacy
Quakertown Hospital

HOW TO USE THIS BOOK

Use this book as a safeguard against medication errors and as a resource guide to drugs that have been associated with some errors.

The 200 errors described in the text actually happened. Some were discovered in time, before patient injury could occur. Others unfortunately ended in tragedy. You can learn from these true stories by studying this book and by sharing them with other nurses.

As you'll discover, the errors are randomly arranged. But you can use this book as a source of reference. Here's how:

Look up possible sources of error in the chart on the following page. It'll direct you to where you can find information on that particular type of error. For example, if you're interested in finding out about drug names that are frequently confused because they're similar-sounding or are similarly written, look in the chart under "Drug name confusion" to find what error numbers the information is in.

You can also use the valuable index at the back of this book to look up certain drug names that have been linked to common medication errors. It's complete with cross references.

TABLE OF ERRORS

SOURCE OF ERROR	ERROR NUMBER
Abbreviation misinterpretation	8, 11, 20, 56, 83, 108, 111, 116, 126, 131, 146, 161, 172, 188, 189, 191
Administration complication	7, 12, 19, 21, 40, 57, 60, 66, 70, 73, 95, 118, 129, 144, 153, 156, 163, 171, 176, 180, 183, 195, 197
Administration route mix-up	24, 100, 114, 138, 155, 188, 194, 196
Allergic reaction	1, 6, 61, 158
Documentation problem	32, 67, 149
Dosage error	5, 13, 17, 18, 28, 33, 35, 43, 49, 50, 53, 55, 72, 77, 81, 97, 105, 108, 119, 133, 141, 149, 154, 157, 163, 181, 192, 193
Drug name confusion	26, 30, 31, 38, 44, 45, 47, 54, 57, 64, 68, 74, 75, 88, 120, 125, 127, 135, 137, 140, 148, 166, 168, 175, 177, 178, 179, 186
Drug preparation problem	25, 67, 76, 89, 92, 120, 145
Equipment misuse	23, 58, 184
Infusion misuse	39, 87, 110, 122
Insulin error	5, 28, 43, 82, 133
I.V. therapy mistake	15, 29, 42, 59, 78, 86, 93, 100, 106, 115, 132, 142, 147, 169
Label confusion	3, 14, 41, 46, 63, 65, 96, 99, 104, 113, 120, 121, 124, 128, 129, 136, 141, 154, 160, 169, 199
MAR misuse	2, 44, 62, 73, 100, 109, 170
Order misunderstanding	22, 79, 80, 85, 101, 123, 130, 134, 143, 150, 159, 182, 190, 200
Patient name mix-up	4, 51, 102, 151, 187
Patient-teaching failure	37, 75
Protocol violation	36, 98
Storage problem	9, 90, 94, 139, 173
Symbol misinterpretation	34, 152
Syringe and Tubex problem	16, 42, 162
Telephone miscommunication	10, 69, 103
Transcription error	2, 52, 81, 185
Unfamiliarity and carelessness	21, 27, 48, 71, 107, 117, 158, 164, 167, 180, 192, 198
Verification failure	20, 53, 84, 91, 112, 165, 174

Not asking yourself, "Is there any reason why the patient shouldn't receive this drug?"

A patient who had arteriosclerotic cardiovascular disease complained to his nurse that he had severe chest pain, unrelieved by nitroglycerin. The nurse notified his doctor, who gave a verbal order for morphine to be given immediately. She quickly prepared and gave the dose. A few minutes later, the nurse transcribed the morphine order to the patient's medication administration record. She glanced at the allergies listed for this patient and was shocked to see morphine as the first allergy on the list.

The nurse rushed to check the patient and call the doctor. Fortunately, the patient suffered no ill effects from the morphine.

You may think that if the patient had been wearing an allergy alert bracelet or had an allergy alert sticker placed over his bed, this error wouldn't have occurred. But these devices *can't* replace deliberate, reasoned thought. Also, don't rely on stickers placed above the bed since patients are often moved without their stickers. Before you administer any drug, you must ask yourself: *Is there any reason why the patient shouldn't receive this drug?* By asking this question, you can consider not only the patient's allergies, but also his condition, which may contraindicate the drug's administration. *Then* you can check for allergy alerts.

So make it a habit. When you check the "five rights" of drug administration (the right patient, drug, dose, time, and route), consider also whether the patient can safely take the drug in the first place. Remember: Bracelets and stickers can't prevent medication errors...but a thinking, vigilant nurse can.

Notes:

Transcribing an order onto the wrong MAR

A doctor wrote an order for Sinemet 10/100 (carbidopa-levodopa) for Mr. Flannery, a patient with Parkinson's disease. That evening, a nurse mistakenly transcribed the order onto the medication administration record (MAR) for Mr. Miller, Mr. Flannery's roommate.

In the meantime, a copy of the doctor's order for Mr. Flannery was sent to the hospital pharmacy. The pharmacist dispensed the Sinemet into Mr. Flannery's bin in the drug cart.

When the medication nurse was ready to administer the drugs, she checked Mr. Miller's MAR, saw the order for Sinemet, and went to his bin in the drug cart to get it. Puzzled that the Sinemet wasn't there, she checked the other bins and found it in Mr. Flannery's. She checked *his* MAR—it had no order for Sinemet.

Thinking the pharmacist had put the Sinemet in the wrong bin, the nurse took the drug from Mr. Flannery's bin and administered it to Mr. Miller. She continued to administer Sinemet to Mr. Miller (taking it from Mr. Flannery's bin) for 2 days.

The error was discovered when Mr. Miller's doctor checked his patient's MAR and saw the order for Sinemet—an order he'd never written. Although Mr. Miller suffered no ill effects from the Sinemet, Mr. Flannery had not received drug therapy for his Parkinson's disease for 2 days.

A mistranscription, an error in judgment, and a lack of drug knowledge contributed to this medication error.

First, the transcribing nurse wrote the order on the wrong MAR—an error that went undiscovered for 2 days. This error could have been prevented if the hospital had a policy of checking the doctor's original order against the patient's MAR within the first 24 hours after an order is written.

Second, the medication nurse switched the drug from one patient's bin to another—defeating a safeguard of the pharmacy's unit-dose system. The nurse should have called the pharmacist when she saw that the drugs in the cart didn't correspond with the patients' MARs.

And third, she could have compared the drug she was administering with the patient's diagnosis. Then she would have questioned why an antiparkinsonism drug was ordered for a patient who didn't have Parkinson's disease.

So if you're responsible for transcribing drug orders, check the name on the MAR first, and be sure you're writing on the right record.

Failing to compare numerically marked tablets with their container's label

While preparing to administer a tablet of Tylenol #3 (acetaminophen, 300 mg, with codeine, 30 mg), a medication nurse noticed the numeral 4 on the tablet. She checked the label on the pharmacy-prepared container and saw it was marked "Tylenol #3." Puzzled, she checked the rest of the tablets in the container—all were imprinted with a numeral 4.

The nurse immediately called the hospital pharmacist to alert him to the discrepancy. He checked his inventory and discovered he'd mistakenly filled all the Tylenol #3 containers with Tylenol #4 tablets (which contain 60 mg of codeine).

By making one last check, this nurse prevented dosage errors for many patients, not just her own. Of course, not all medications are numerically coded, so you can't always compare them with the container's label. But when you *can* compare, do so. That extra check just might prevent a medication error.

Notes:
_____
_____
_____
_____
_____

Error
Number

4

Assuming the name "Wright" to be an affirmative reply

A nurse was relieving the regular medication nurse on a tuberculosis ward. All went well until she asked a patient, "Are you Mr. Thomas?" "Wright," he answered.

Assuming the patient had given an affirmative reply, the nurse then gave Mr. Wright the medications intended for Mr. Thomas. She realized her error two patients later when she found the *real* Mr. Thomas. Fortunately, since both men were receiving the same medication and dosage, no harm was done. Mr. Wright, however, also received a dose of clorazepate dipotassium (Tranxene) intended for Mr. Thomas.

Misidentifying a patient is one of the most common causes of medication errors. And checking a patient's identification band is the only sure way to identify him, although it may seem to be a bother. Even when you think you know your patient by sight, a last-minute transfer from one room to another, a confused patient, or similar-sounding patient names could lead to misidentification.

So always check the patient's identification band before administering a medication—and if he doesn't have one, get him one before you continue your rounds.

Notes:

Drawing up insulin in a tuberculin syringe and failing to have another nurse double-check the dose

A brittle diabetic patient being treated for ketoacidosis was transferred from the intensive care unit to a medical/surgical floor. A new graduate nurse checked the patient's orders: He was to receive 9 units of NPH insulin at 4:30 p.m.

Since the unit was temporarily out of insulin syringes, the nurse decided to use a 1-ml tuberculin syringe instead. This syringe was graded in tenths of a milliliter, and since U-100 insulin was being used, she thought she could determine the correct dose. She drew up the insulin to the 0.9 ml mark and administered the injection.

The patient ate poorly at dinnertime. Around 8 p.m., the nurse noted he was groggy and sweaty. She called a doctor, who immediately ordered a blood glucose level measurement—it showed extreme hypoglycemia. He injected 100 ml of 50% dextrose solution, and the patient gradually recovered. But not until the next day did the nurse realize that 0.9 ml of U-100 insulin drawn up in the tuberculin syringe equaled *ninety* units, not nine.

This nurse learned the hard way two cardinal rules for administering insulin: (1) Use only an insulin syringe to draw up and administer insulin, and (2) have another nurse double-check the dose you've drawn up. If the hospital pharmacist has prepared a unit-dose syringe of insulin, double-check *his* work.

Notes:

_____

_____

_____

_____

_____

Error Number	**Forgetting to check for a patient's drug allergies**
6	

A nursing instructor on clinical rounds with her students checked the Kardex and spotted a new order for an intramuscular (I.M.) injection of penicillin. Since her students needed experience administering I.M. injections, she decided this patient would afford a good opportunity to test their skills.

The instructor assigned a student to give the injection, and together they checked the patient's medication administration record (MAR) against the doctor's original order, written on the patient's chart. They also went over the five "rights" of medication administration—right patient, right drug, right dose, right time, and right route. Everything seemed to check out, so the student gave the injection.

The patient, enjoying all this attention, asked what the injection was. When the student said it was penicillin, he said quietly, "But I'm allergic to penicillin."

The instructor immediately rechecked the chart and MAR. Although the allergy was noted on the patient's health history, neither the chart nor the MAR had been flagged with an allergy alert.

The patient developed a rash and facial swelling from the penicillin, and was given 50 mg of diphenhydramine HCl (Benadryl) I.M. to counteract these effects.

The instructor used this incident to make several points about checking for allergies:

1. When you compare the patient's MAR with the doctor's original order, also check the chart for allergies.

2. If the patient is allergic to a drug, be sure an allergy alert appears both on the MAR and on the *front* of the chart.

3. Suggest the patient get an armband to identify his allergy.

4. Before administering drugs that frequently cause allergic reactions (e.g., antibiotics, narcotics, aspirin), ask the patient if there are any medications he can't take.

The hospital can also provide an additional safeguard: Many pharmacies maintain drug profiles that include each patient's diagnosis and allergies. The pharmacist compares all new orders with the profile, and so provides still another check for possible drug allergies.

Leaving substances at a patient's bedside without giving clear instructions

A patient who'd just had a pacemaker implanted was to have his incision cleaned with hydrogen peroxide. His nurse poured some peroxide into a medicine cup and set it on the patient's bedside table, saying, "Here's your hydrogen peroxide—I'll be right back." Then she left the room to get some gauze pads.

When she returned a few minutes later, the cup was empty. The patient, thinking it was medicine, had swallowed the hydrogen peroxide. The nurse called the doctor, who decided an antidote was unnecessary. The patient complained of a burning mouth and stomachache but was otherwise unharmed. However, he was so upset by the incident that his family transferred him to another hospital.

The lesson is clear: A disinfectant, antiseptic, soap, or other substance left at the bedside in a medicine cup can easily be mistaken for a medication. Usually, you shouldn't leave *any* substances (including medications) at the bedside. But if you must leave something (e.g., an antiseptic or soap for a patient doing his own wound care), be sure you also give him clear explanations of what it is and how to use it.

Notes:
_____
_____
_____
_____
_____

Using "sub q" for subcutaneously instead of "s.c."

A patient scheduled for an abdominal hysterectomy was admitted to an obstetric unit because the surgical unit was being renovated. The evening before surgery, the surgeon, who routinely ordered heparin prophylactically for his patients, wrote this order:

heparin 5,000 units sub q2h prior to surgery

The obstetric nurses, who weren't familiar with the surgeon's routine, interpreted the order as "heparin, 5,000 units, subcutaneously, every 2 hours prior to surgery." Although the nurses and their supervisor questioned the high dosage, they didn't call the doctor. They gave the patient 5,000 units of heparin every 2 hours throughout the night.

At the morning change of shift, the oncoming supervisor also questioned the order. But when she checked the patient's chart, she interpreted the order differently (and as the doctor had intended): 5,000 units of heparin to be given subcutaneously 2 hours before surgery.

The supervisor quickly notified the doctor. He canceled the surgery and ordered laboratory tests, which showed a prolonged activated partial thromboplastin time (PTT). He rescheduled the surgery for the following day, and the patient withstood it with no complications.

This dangerous and costly error could have been prevented if the doctor had used "s.c."—the accepted abbreviation for "subcutaneously"—instead of "sub q." The nurses who read his order saw "sub q2h" not "sub q 2h" and interpreted the "q" as "every." And though they *did* question the order, they didn't call the doctor or a pharmacist or check a drug reference, which would have confirmed that 5,000 units of heparin every 2 hours is a most unusual order.

So when you transcribe an order for a subcutaneous injection, use the accepted abbreviation. If you see "sub q" written on an order, look closer. You may spot an error in the making.

Neglecting to check with the pharmacist if a drug choice looks incorrect

A severely burned patient had a continuing order for 50 mg of diphenhydramine HCl (Benadryl) to relieve itching. After several weeks of administering this drug, most of the unit nurses were familiar with it.

But one day, when a nurse took the patient's unit dose of medication from his bin in the medication cart, she thought it looked different—more like dimenhydrinate (Dramamine) than diphenhydramine. The package label confirmed her suspicion: It *was* phenytoin.

The nurse checked the patient's chart to see if a new order had been written for the dimenhydrinate. Finding none, she notified the pharmacist of the discrepancy.

The pharmacist remembered refilling the order for diphenhydramine but was unaware that the wrong drug had been dispensed. When the nurse asked him if these two medications could have been mixed up in his supply, he realized what had happened.

These two drugs were stored side by side on the pharmacy shelf. The pharmacist realized that when he had dispensed the drug, he'd apparently read the shelf labels of the drugs too quickly. Because their names were so similar, he accidentally reached for the wrong one.

In this case, a nurse's thoroughness and persistence prevented a medication error. Many nurses, however, assume that whatever drug is in the patient's bin must be the right drug to give him—especially when they've become comfortable with the unit-dose system. But pharmacist error can cause the system to break down. That's why you still must read the package label and compare it with the medication administration record before administering a drug from a medication cart bin. If something doesn't look right, check the original order. Then question the pharmacist.

Notes:

_____

_____

_____

_____

_____

Error
Number

10

Not clarifying laboratory test results given by telephone

A diabetic patient underwent surgery and was sent to the recovery room with an order for a stat blood glucose. The recovery room nurse drew the blood sample and sent it to the laboratory.

Later, when she called the laboratory for the test result, the technician said "442." The nurse repeated "442?" The technician said yes, and hung up. The nurse then called the surgeon and gave him the same number. He, in turn, ordered insulin for the patient.

Just before she added the insulin to the patient's I.V., the nurse got a call from the same technician. "Something's been bothering me about your phone call," he said. "Did I tell you the test result was 442?" The nurse said yes. "Well," said the technician, "I meant for you to *call extension 442* to get the result."

The nurse called the extension, found that the patient's blood glucose level was 90 mg/100 ml (within normal limits), and had the insulin order canceled.

In a similar incident, a nurse requested a stat blood glucose test for Mr. Jones, the patient in Room 315. When the technician called back with the result, he said, "I have the blood glucose result on Mr. Jones, 315." The busy nurse wrote down 315, said thanks, and abruptly hung up.

She then told the patient's doctor the blood glucose level was 315. The doctor ordered insulin, and in this case, the nurse administered it. When she received the written laboratory report later, she discovered her error: Mr. Jones's blood glucose level was actually 650 mg/100 ml. She called the doctor, who ordered an additional dose of insulin.

Luckily, neither of these patients suffered any harm. But the nurses and technicians learned the value of clarifying test results taken or given by telephone.

You can avoid a similar mistake by repeating back the information you've just been given; for example, "You say that Mr. Jones's blood glucose level is 315 mg/100 ml?" That extra precaution won't take extra time, but it will prevent misinterpreting those crucial laboratory test results.

Using the abbreviation "q.d." for daily

A patient with a diagnosis of middle cerebral artery thrombosis was admitted to a medical unit. Because the patient couldn't speak, his son gave the admitting nurse the medical history, including medications the patient was taking. The nurse attached the list of medications and their dosages to the front of the patient's chart and handed it to the doctor.

Later that evening, the nurse reviewed the medication orders the doctor had written for this patient. She was surprised to see an order for digoxin (Lanoxin), 0.25 mg, q.i.d., when she clearly remembered the patient's son saying his father took Lanoxin only once a day. So she looked at the doctor's order again, confirmed that it said q.i.d., and transcribed it onto the medication Kardex.

Because the nurse was new on the unit, she asked the charge nurse to check the orders she'd transcribed. When the charge nurse saw the Lanoxin order, she too questioned it. Both nurses examined the doctor's written order again...and agreed it said q.i.d. Nevertheless, the charge nurse was uncomfortable with the increased dosage and called the doctor for verification.

The doctor claimed he wrote q.d.—once daily—not q.i.d. But his order looked like this.

The period after the "q" looked exactly like an "i."

Luckily for the patient, the order was corrected before a dose was given. If he'd received Lanoxin four times a day, he'd have developed digoxin toxicity and could have died.

This near-error could have been avoided if the doctor had written out the word *daily* on the medication order instead of using the abbreviation q.d. This is an unacceptable abbreviation. But the nurse compounded the doctor's error by transcribing what she knew was an unusually high dosage.

To avoid similar errors, be sure you know the dosages of the drugs you administer. Don't hesitate to ask the doctor to verify unusually high dosages. And work to eliminate the use of the abbreviation q.d. for daily.

Error
Number

12

Administering a drug without being sure it corresponds with the patient's diagnosis

A nurse on a medical unit went to check on an elderly man who'd been treated for a small stasis ulcer and was scheduled for discharge the next day. When she assessed him, she found him unresponsive to painful stimuli, pale, diaphoretic, and with a weak, thready pulse. Immediately, she called the doctor.

At first, the doctor thought the patient had developed a pulmonary embolism. Then the nurse remembered, "He got his first dose of Tolinase (tolazamide) this morning."

Because the patient wasn't diabetic, the doctor denied ordering tolazamide, an oral hypoglycemic agent. But the nurse showed him his handwritten order on the patient's chart. Then the doctor realized what had happened: He'd meant to write the order for a different patient, but had mixed up the two patients' charts.

The doctor diagnosed the elderly patient as having developed hypoglycemia from the tolazamide and ordered intravenous glucose. The patient's condition rapidly returned to normal.

This potentially life-threatening error could have been prevented if the doctor had been more careful when writing his orders, and by double-checking the patient's name and room number on the front of the chart and the order sheet.

But equally important, the nurse who administered the tolazamide should have questioned why a hypoglycemic agent was ordered for a patient who didn't have diabetes. If she'd asked the doctor before administering the drug, she would have prevented the error.

So know your patient's diagnosis and the indication for the drug you're about to give. If the two don't agree, check with the doctor to make sure the order's correct.

Notes:

Calculating doses in your head—not on paper

In his third week after a cholecystectomy, a patient developed a fistula and his temperature spiked to 102° F. (38.9° C.). The attending doctor ordered 1.5 million (1,500,000) units of intravenous penicillin G potassium to be given every 4 hours.

The pharmacist dispensed four vials of the penicillin, each labeled 5,000,000 (5 million) units...the smallest containers of this drug the pharmacy had in stock. He intended the vials to be given over 2 days.

When the medication nurse was ready to administer the penicillin, she mentally calculated, "The order is for 1.5 million units; 5 plus 5 plus 5 equals 1.5 million." Then she took three of the vials from the patient's bin, added them to a solution of D_5W, and piggybacked the solution into the patient's primary infusion.

When she was charting what she'd administered, she casually mentioned to another nurse, "We'll have to order more penicillin for Mr. Lanford. We have only one vial left."

The second nurse had seen the four vials when they were delivered and knew they were more than enough for one dose. So she asked the medication nurse what she had given the patient. Immediately, the medication nurse realized that by calculating quickly in her head, she'd misplaced a decimal point. Instead of giving 1.5 million units, she'd given 15 million units.

The nurse called the doctor right away, and they both checked the patient. Although the drug had completely infused, the patient was not harmed. But the doctor ordered all other doses of penicillin withheld through the night.

To avoid making similar errors, always calculate doses on paper, not in your head. Then you'll be sure all decimal points are placed correctly. Also, read vial labels carefully, especially if large amounts—written with several zeros—are involved.

Finally, recheck your calculations if you must use several vials or ampules to prepare one dose. Usually, this is a clue that you're preparing too much medication.

Notes:

_____

_____

_____

_____

_____

Misinterpreting a manufacturer's package label

A doctor ordered 650 mg of buffered aspirin three times a day for a patient with arthritis. When the nurse on afternoon medication rounds checked the patient's bin of the medication cart, she saw two 2-tablet unit-dose packages of this product. She compared the drug order with the package label, which listed the dose as "aspirin, 325 mg...."

The nurse assumed that the label on a unit-dose package described the total package contents. Because the label didn't state "325 mg per single tablet" or "each tablet contains 325 mg," she assumed the entire package contained 325 mg. So she administered two entire packages (4 tablets) to the patient, thinking she was giving 650 mg.

After completing rounds, the nurse told the pharmacist she'd need more packages for the evening dose. The pharmacist was sure he'd put enough medication for the day in the patient's bin, so he asked her how many packages she'd given the patient. When she told him, he explained that *each tablet* in the package contains 325 mg, so a 2-tablet package contains 650 mg.

Luckily, the patient wasn't harmed by this double dose of aspirin. But he could have developed aspirin toxicity if the error had been repeated indefinitely.

Although the nurse knew that most aspirin tablets contain 325 mg, she interpreted the package label literally and didn't ask the pharmacist to confirm her interpretation. And she didn't ask herself why she was giving two packages for one dose—often a clue that something is wrong. Nevertheless, the package label *was* misleading.

The nurse, upset by her error, decided to take action. She wrote to the drug manufacturer, explained what had happened, and pointed out that the label on a 2-tablet package of a similar product states "each tablet contains 325 mg." A few months later, the manufacturer agreed to revise the label.

If you have a similar problem with a package label, report it in a detailed letter to the manufacturer.

Also, you can notify either the United States Pharmacopeia (USP) Drug Product Problem-Reporting Program or the FDA. The USP will investigate the complaint and contact the manufacturer. Call the Drug Product Problem-Reporting Program toll-free at (800) 638-6725 between 9 a.m. and 4:30 p.m. on weekdays. (At other times, a recording device takes your complaint.) In Maryland, Hawaii, and Alaska, call collect (301) 881-0256 between 9 a.m. and 4:40 p.m. weekdays.

Using macrodrip tubing instead of microdrip

A continuous infusion of aminophylline, 40 mg per hour, was ordered for an elderly man with asthma. The nurse prepared a concentration of 1 gram of aminophylline in 250 ml D_5W (40 mg per 10 ml) and hung the bottle. She then attached a nonvolumetric (drop-counting) infusion controller (not to be confused with an infusion pump) to the intravenous tubing.

At change of shift, the nurse mentioned in report that more than 200 ml of solution remained in the bottle, enough to last well through the next two shifts. But at the end of the second shift, another nurse noticed that the I.V. bottle was empty. She quickly checked the controller; it was set at 10 drops per minute (the correct rate for a microdrip I.V. set that delivers 60 drops per ml). Then she discovered that the infusion was flowing through *macro*drip tubing, which delivers 20 drops per ml. As a result, the patient was receiving 30 ml per hour instead of the prescribed 10 ml per hour.

The nurse called the doctor, who ordered the infusion discontinued and blood drawn for analysis. The patient complained of severe nausea, a result of the aminophylline overdose.

This error was not the fault of the machine but rather of the user. A drop-counting infusion controller is a precision instrument when used correctly. But because it accommodates any size I.V. tubing, errors like this one can occur.

To avoid similar errors, be sure you understand completely how a drop-counting controller works. Make sure you attach the correct size tubing.

Check the drip rate visually to see if it's running too fast; don't rely only on the controller. Time-taping the I.V. bottle can help you monitor the rate.

Ask your pharmacist to prepare a chart showing the correct flow rates and tubing to be used for standard concentrations of frequently infused drugs. Keep the chart handy for easy reference.

Volumetric gravity-dependent rate controllers are set in ml per hour, not drops per minute. This controller eliminates the need for calculating a drop rate. Also, only the tubing specifically intended for the machine can be attached to it.

<table>
<tr><td>

Error
Number

16

</td><td>

Confusing two different types of lidocaine syringes

</td></tr>
</table>

During a routine surgical procedure, a patient developed premature ventricular contractions. The anesthesiologist told the circulating nurse to administer a bolus of 100 mg of lidocaine (lignocaine) through an injection port on the patient's I.V. line. He removed the prefilled syringe from its box and handed it to her. The nurse injected the drug into the infusing I.V. line, and injected a second dose a few minutes later at the anesthesiologist's request.

Soon after the two doses had been injected, another operating room (OR) nurse picked up the empty syringes and saw they were labeled: "lidocaine, *1 gram*. CAUTION: MUST BE DILUTED." The patient had received 2 *grams* of lidocaine rather than the 200 mg intended.

After surgery, the patient was closely monitored, and he survived the accidental overdose. But he was lucky; similar mix-ups between 100-mg and 1-gram lidocaine syringes have caused death.

Why did this potentially fatal medication error occur? Two factors contributed to it.

First is the confusion inherent in having two types of lidocaine prefilled syringes available. One type, containing either 50 or 100 mg, is intended for I.V. bolus injection. The second type (the one accidentally injected in this incident) contains either 1 or 2 grams of the drug. These syringes are intended for preparing large-volume dilutions of lidocaine for continuous infusion.

The 1- and 2-gram syringes, manufactured by several companies, contain concentrated lidocaine. This type of syringe has a very short needle, which allows it to be used as a universal additive syringe. In other words, you can use it to add the drug to a glass I.V. bottle, through the rubber stopper, or to an I.V. bag, through its injection port.

The universal additive syringes look quite different from syringes meant for bolus injections—a bulbous cap covers most of the needle. Also, they're clearly marked CAUTION: MUST BE DILUTED. But the needle does stick out far enough from the cap to fit into an injection port or intermittent infusion (INT) device.

The second contributing factor is that some hospitals routinely stock both types of syringes in the OR on crash carts and on nursing units. This practice can lead to confusion in an emergency. True—the boxes in which they're packaged have different colors. But in this incident, a doctor removed a syringe from its box and handed it to a nurse to administer. The nurse didn't see the box. And hurrying to administer the drug, she didn't take time to read the syringe's label, assuming that the doctor had checked it.

Avoid stocking concentrated lidocaine syringes at all. Vials of concentrate with transfer sets are available; and recently, three manufacturers of large volume parenterals have introduced pre-mixed solutions of lidocaine in glass and plastic containers—ready to infuse. Consider discussing these alternatives with your hospital pharmacist.

Notes:

Error Number	Assuming an order for

Error Number

17

Assuming an order for cancer chemotherapeutic drugs is correct

A nurse working the day shift prepared to administer medication to the 50 patients on her medical unit. A medication administration record (MAR) written the evening before for an 80-pound (36-kg) woman with breast cancer had this order:

Adriamycin 150 mg, Cytoxan, 1500 mg (on floor).

Because the nurse didn't know what "on floor" meant, she asked her head nurse. The head nurse explained it meant to have the drugs available so the intern could give them...and she reminded the medication nurse that only doctors could give I.V. chemotherapeutic drugs.

Because the doses of Adriamycin (doxorubicin HCl) and Cytoxan (cyclophosphamide) seemed high for this small patient, the nurse checked the MAR against the doctor's original order. The transcription was correct, so she got the drugs from the pharmacy.

When she returned, she found the intern and said, "Here are the drugs for you to give Mrs. Smith. Nurses don't give I.V. chemotherapy." She then watched the intern prepare the medication and administer it—*all* of it—to the patient.

That evening, the patient's doctor came to the unit and asked for the medication he had ordered the evening before. The intern told him he had administered the entire dose of both drugs to the patient.

The astonished doctor quickly checked his patient. Because of his concern that her blood cell count would drop drastically, he placed her in reverse isolation for the next 2 weeks. She had a fever, suffered severe nausea and vomiting, and eventually needed numerous blood transfusions. Fortunately, she didn't develop cardiotoxicity, which can result from an overdose of Adriamycin.

The patient was lucky to bear this high dose of highly toxic drugs. Nevertheless, all involved in the error were horrified by it—especially the nurse, who was blamed for the error.

Actually, several errors were made. First, the patient's doctor wrote an incomplete order. He didn't specify that he wanted the drugs on the floor so he could give them in *divided* doses over several days. He also neglected to specify time and route of administration.

The nurse, though she thought the doses seemed high, assumed that because the doctor was an expert in oncology, the order was correct. She also assumed the intern was familiar with the protocol for administering the drugs. The head nurse added to the confusion by not questioning the order herself.

The pharmacist compounded the error by dispensing an incomplete order. Finally, the intern administered the drugs in one dose without checking the protocol and because he thought the medication nurse had told him to do it.

All these people contributed to the error by not checking with the prescribing doctor to confirm that the order was correct. Each assumed the other knew what he was doing.

Obviously, you should never assume anything when you're responsible for medication administration. But for highly toxic cancer drugs, still more safeguards are needed in hospital policies and procedures.

For example, the hospital could require that all chemotherapy orders be written during the day, when a full staff of doctors, nurses, and pharmacists are available to double-check them. The hospital could post its chemotherapy protocols on each nursing unit. Or it could establish a cancer chemotherapy unit and require that everyone on this unit be familiar with the drugs' protocols.

Whatever the policy in the hospital where you work, remember: When you're working with cancer drugs, *you're* responsible for their safe administration. If the drug order seems unclear, don't assume it's correct—confirm it with the prescribing doctor.

Notes:

Error
Number

18

Not listening to your patient if he questions his medication or the dosage

A student nurse drew up 85 units of NPH insulin for a diabetic patient, as ordered on the patient's medication Kardex. But when she and her instructor approached the patient to administer the insulin, he protested that there was too much in the syringe. When the student explained that an order had been written for 85 units, the patient refused the injection, saying his usual dose was 10 units each morning.

Immediately, the student and instructor checked the patient's medication Kardex and the doctor's original order. Both specified 85 units. Then they called the patient's doctor—who told them the patient was correct. The doctor immediately changed the order to 10 units of NPH insulin every morning.

Hoping to get to the root of the error, the nursing instructor checked with the doctor who'd been on call the night before, when the patient was admitted. This doctor explained that he'd taken the order for 85 units from the patient's chart for his last admission—a year before. Apparently, he never asked the patient whether his insulin requirements had changed since the last admission. Nor did he check with the patient's regular doctor.

By listening to the patient, these nurses prevented a dangerous medication error. Too often, a patient's questions about his medication are not taken seriously. Yet patients are becoming more aware of the need to know what they're taking. And their knowledge has become increasingly important in preventing medication errors.

So *listen* to your patient. If he says the dose looks too large or his usual pills are a different color, hold the dose and confirm the order with his doctor.

And take every opportunity to encourage a patient to be a careful health consumer. Teach him his drugs' names, what they're used for, what they look like, and his usual dosage of each. When you administer a drug, say something like "Here's your daily dose of NPH insulin for your diabetes—10 units." That way, the patient will become familiar with his drugs and will be more likely to question a different tablet or a changed dose.

Leaving nitroglycerin ointment within a patient's reach

A nursing supervisor making rounds at a convalescent center entered the area for confused patients. She noticed a tube of nitroglycerin ointment on top of a unit-dose cart. No nurse was in sight.

She waited for the medication nurse to return, then reminded her that *all* medications must be kept inside the cart when it was unattended. The nurse promised she would lock up the ointment as soon as she finished using it.

Later that morning, the medication nurse called her supervisor and said, "I learned my lesson! I've looked everywhere for that ointment. Now tell me where you hid it." Unfortunately, the supervisor *hadn't* hidden it...and she had no idea where it was.

The staff quickly searched each room and finally found the ointment with an elderly patient. She said she'd taken the "skin cream" to soothe the dry skin on her legs. The nurses quickly wiped off the ointment.

The nitroglycerin ointment could have severely lowered her blood pressure possibly causing her to fall. Even a small amount can cause dizziness and severe headaches.

Preventing this kind of error is easy: Never leave medications within patient reach when you're not there. As soon as you've finished using a drug, lock it up.

Notes: _____

_____

_____

_____

_____

Error Number

20

Discontinuing medication without checking with the doctor first

A community health nurse received a hospital care plan for a new home-care patient that had the following orders:

> Tentative dscharge in Am tomorrow
> D/C meds : Coumadin 5 mg PO daily

Interpreting "D/C" to mean *discontinue,* the nurse wondered why warfarin sodium (Coumadin) would be discontinued for this patient, who had a history of strokes. The nurse tried calling the doctor to question the order. When she couldn't reach him, she decided to tell the patient to stop taking the Coumadin.

Several weeks later, the patient returned to the hospital clinic for a prothrombin time test. When the test result showed no anti-coagulant effect, the doctor asked him if he had stopped taking Coumadin. The patient replied that the community health nurse had told him to discontinue it.

The puzzled doctor called the nurse. When she explained that the care plan said to "D/C the med," the doctor realized what had happened. He had used D/C to mean *discharge,* intending that the medication be taken after the patient left the hospital.

The patient's Coumadin regimen was immediately restarted. Although not taking the anticoagulant hadn't harmed him, a blood clot could have formed.

To prevent such an error, avoid using D/C when referring to medications to be taken by a discharged patient. Warn your colleagues to do the same, and write out "discharge" and "discontinue" on orders.

Notes:

_____

_____

_____

_____

_____

Leaving medications for a patient to take later

A nurse in an extended-care facility knew her patients well enough to know she could trust some of them to take their medications unsupervised. One night, she left a patient's evening medications on his bedside table when he was out of his room, because she knew he'd take them when he returned.

The nurse completed her medication rounds and began her charting. A little later, a nursing assistant appeared at the nurses' station with a patient from another floor.

"Mr. Jones decided to visit your floor," the nursing assistant explained, "and while he was here, he went into a patient's room and took the medications on the bedside table. We're trying to find out what they were."

The nurse realized immediately whose medications Mr. Jones had taken. She quickly called the doctor and reported the incident. The doctor ordered that Mr. Jones be closely monitored for the next 24 hours. Luckily, he suffered no ill effects from the drugs.

This medication error occurred because a nurse—with the best intentions—bent one of the rules of safe drug administration: Never leave drugs for a patient to take on his own—stay with him until you *observe* him take them.

Leaving medications for a patient to take later could lead to any number of problems. For instance, a patient may decide to skip a dose. The patient's roommate may take the drugs by mistake. Or even more frightening, a depressed patient may hoard sedatives or other drugs and later take them all at once in a suicide attempt.

To prevent such errors, don't leave medications for a patient to take later, unless the drugs are specifically ordered for self-administration (e.g., nitroglycerin, antacids). Stay and observe the patient take his drugs. If he refuses a dose, make a note of it and take the drug with you. If it's a p.r.n. medication or bedtime sedative, return later and offer the drug again.

Notes:

_____

_____

_____

_____

_____

Error Number

22

Not writing a zero before a decimal point on medication orders

A patient suffering an acute asthma attack was admitted to a busy emergency department (ED). The ED doctor prescribed, among other things, 0.5 mg of the bronchodilator terbutaline (Brethine, Bricanyl).

Because the ED order sheet had so much written on it, the doctor had to squeeze in his order for terbutaline. He wrote it like this:

Terbutaline .5 mg now SQ

Although the decimal point was hard to see, the ED nurses were familiar with the drug and administered the correct dose.

The patient's condition improved in the ED, but the doctor decided to admit him to the hospital for observation. Another doctor, called in to write the admitting orders, simply copied the orders from the ED order sheet. Not noticing the decimal point in front of the 5 in the terbutaline order, he wrote 5 mg as the dose.

The patient and his admission orders were transferred to a medical floor. There, the nurse transcribing the orders asked the admitting doctor if he really meant to give the patient 5 mg of terbutaline. The doctor replied, "I wrote the order, didn't I?" So the nurse drew up 5 mg of terbutaline and administered it to the patient.

Within 10 minutes, the patient developed hypertension, tachycardia, and a pounding headache from this injection—which was *10* times what he should have received. He had to be moved to the intensive care unit, where he spent 2 days recovering from the overdose.

Several factors led to this medication error. Most important, the ED doctor should have written a zero before the decimal point in his order. In the cramped space on the order sheet, the decimal point virtually disappeared.

Second, the admitting doctor shouldn't have copied the orders without fully understanding them. And when the transcribing nurse questioned his order for 5 mg, he should have listened to her concerns.

Third, the transcribing nurse shouldn't have let the doctor's abrupt attitude deter her from checking the correct dosage range for terbutaline herself, either with another colleague or in a drug reference. Obviously, she knew something was wrong with the order, so she shouldn't have carried it out until she was satisfied it was correct.

Abbreviating an order to fit it onto a crowded order sheet may seem like a good idea. But in this incident, the squeezed-in order seriously harmed a patient. So starting now, make it a habit to *always* write a zero before a decimal point on medication order transcriptions. You'll definitely save confusion about the dose, and you may just save a patient's life.

Notes:

_____

_____

_____

_____

_____

Error
Number

23

Failing to clean the mortar and pestle after crushing tablets

During the evening shift, a medication nurse used a mortar and pestle to crush a penicillin tablet for one of her patients. When she went off duty, she left the mortar and pestle on top of the drug cart without cleaning them.

On the next shift, another nurse used the same mortar and pestle to crush a tablet for a different patient. Immediately after she administered the crushed tablet, the patient became dyspneic and cyanotic and lost consciousness. The nurse called a code and the patient was successfully resuscitated.

After the crisis was over, the nurse found out that the mortar and pestle hadn't been cleaned after their last use—crushing a penicillin tablet. The tiny bit of penicillin left in the mortar was mixed with the tablet she was crushing. It was enough to put this patient, who was severely allergic to penicillin, into anaphylactic shock.

This error could have been prevented if the mortar and pestle had been thoroughly cleaned after their use. But an even better way to prevent this type of error is to check first with a pharmacist before crushing any tablets.

Many medications today are issued in sustained-release or enteric-coated tablets. If you crush a sustained-release tablet, you'll destroy its long-acting effect. In other words, the patient will get the entire dose all at once instead of over a period of hours. Crushing an enteric-coated tablet causes the drug to be released before it should be, in the stomach rather than the small intestine.

Obviously, you shouldn't crush these tablets. If a patient can't swallow a tablet whole, ask the pharmacist whether a liquid form of the drug is available. If not, the pharmacist may be able to prepare a special formulation or suggest an alternative.

Notes:

_____

_____

_____

_____

_____

Forgetting to check
the administration route

A nurse working the night shift read this medication order for a woman recovering from a cerebral vascular accident:

Mycostatin suppository, one at bedtime

The nurse prepared a Mycostatin (nystatin) vaginal tablet according to its package instructions and inserted it into the patient's vagina.

The following morning, the oncoming supervisor asked the nurse if she had given the patient her suppository vaginally. The nurse said yes, but sensing something was amiss asked, "Is anything wrong?"

The supervisor replied, "Well, the patient was supposed to dissolve the drug in her mouth. She has an *oral* yeast infection." The nurse immediately checked the patient's medication Kardex. Sure enough, next to the order were the letters *P.O. and "dissolve in mouth."*

The patient suffered no ill effects from receiving the Mycostatin vaginally, although she missed out on a dose to treat her infection. So even when a drug's administration route seems obvious, check it against the medication Kardex anyway. You may prevent an error—*and* save yourself and your patient some embarrassment.

Notes:

| Error Number | **Allowing yourself to be distracted while preparing drugs** |

25

An emergency department nurse received an order for 0.3 ml of subcutaneous epinephrine to treat an asthmatic patient and went to the drug supply room to get it. Because storage space was limited there, several different medications, including ampules of epinephrine (Adrenalin), benztropine mesylate (Cogentin), and haloperidol (Haldol) were stored in the same drawer.

As the nurse reached for the epinephrine, an X-ray technician who was leaving for the day stopped by to say good night. The two talked while the nurse drew up the medication.

The nurse then went to the examining room where the patient was waiting and administered the injection. She returned to the supply room to discard the used medication ampule. But when she picked it up, she was shocked to see it was not epinephrine but benztropine, an anticholinergic.

The nurse quickly notified the doctor, who told her to administer the epinephrine anyway. As it turned out, the benztropine didn't harm the patient.

The nurse was quite shaken by the incident. She realized how easily she could be distracted—and how dangerous that could be when preparing medications.

Never let anyone or anything distract you when you're preparing a drug for administration. If someone needs to talk to you, ask him to wait until you've administered the drug. And be sure to practice what you learned in nursing school...to check the drug label at least three times: (1) when you remove the drug from a supply drawer or medication cart, (2) before you administer it to the patient, and (3) before you discard its container.

Notes:

_____

_____

_____

_____

_____

Giving camphorated oil instead of castor oil

A doctor scheduled an outpatient for a barium enema and told the man to take 2 ounces (60 ml) of castor oil the evening before the procedure. The man's daughter, a nurse, bought the oil at a neighborhood pharmacy, then went right home and gave it to her father. The man, remembering how he'd hated castor oil as a child, swallowed the dose quickly.

Immediately, the man said he felt a burning sensation in his stomach. His daughter looked more closely at the bottle's label. To her horror, she saw that it was not castor oil but *20% camphorated oil,* a rubbing compound that can be fatal if ingested.

The daughter rushed her father to an emergency department, where gastric lavage was performed. The man was closely observed throughout the night, and he recovered with no ill effects.

The next day, the man's daughter returned to the pharmacy where she had bought the oil to see how she had picked up the wrong bottle. She found that the castor oil was placed on a shelf directly above the camphorated oil. Both bottles were the same size, made of clear glass, with similar blue-striped labels. She told the pharmacist what had happened, and he agreed that the two products should be separated.

As you know, many drug labels look alike. To avoid confusing drugs as this nurse did, read labels carefully, regardless of whether you're taking a medication from a hospital supply room or from a neighborhood pharmacy or supermarket shelf.

To help prevent a similar error outside the hospital, take every opportunity to teach your patients, family, and friends the importance of reading a label carefully before taking a drug themselves or administering it to someone else.

Ironically, this nurse's father may have been the last person to accidentally ingest camphorated oil. After a 6-year campaign, a New Jersey community pharmacist convinced the Food and Drug Administration to withdraw camphorated oil (a product with little or no therapeutic value) from the market.

Notes:

Failing to look up an unfamiliar drug before administering it

A 35-year-old man underwent an appendectomy. About 4 hours after the operation, he told his nurse he was unable to urinate. The nurse examined him and found that his bladder was distended. Although the doctor had left an order for straight catheterization, the patient refused to be catheterized.

The nurse notified the doctor, who then ordered an intramuscular injection of neostigmine (Prostigmin), a cholinergic that stimulates bladder contraction while relaxing the bladder sphincter. Unfortunately, the doctor made two mistakes in writing that order. First, he overlooked the patient's history of asthma. Cholinergics can cause bronchoconstriction in asthmatic patients, precipitating an acute asthmatic attack.

Second, the doctor ordered a dose of 25 mg instead of the correct dose of 0.25 mg. The nurse, unfamiliar with neostigmine, transcribed the order exactly as written. Then she went to the unit supply room to prepare the dose. There, she obtained a 10-ml vial containing a 1:2,000 solution of neostigmine.

The nurse calculated (incorrectly) that she'd need 5 ml of the solution to equal 25 mg of neostigmine. (The correct calculation would have been 50 ml.) But she prepared the injection of 5 ml and administered it to the patient. Since she didn't know how quickly the drug acts, she didn't leave a bedpan or the call bell within his reach. Then she continued on her medication rounds.

Some 15 minutes later, the nurse checked on the patient. She found a trail of urine and blood leading to his bathroom.

In his urgency to get there, the patient had climbed over the side rails and dislodged his intravenous catheter. He was barely able to stand; his face was flushed; he was wheezing and short of breath; he was incontinent; and he complained of incisional pain and severe abdominal cramps. The nurse called for help and another nurse quickly called the doctor. He ordered atropine, an anticholinergic, to reverse the effects of neostigmine. After a miserable night, the patient fully recovered from the overdose.

This series of errors drastically compounded the patient's misery. The doctor broke a cardinal rule for prescribing a cholinergic: Check first for asthma. If the doctor had been aware of the patient's asthma, he probably wouldn't have ordered the drug but rather would have emphasized to the patient the necessity of catheterization. Instead, he ordered a 100-fold overdose.

The nurse added to the error by not checking a drug she wasn't familiar with before administering it. If she had looked up neostigmine in a reference book, she'd have found it was not recommended for patients with asthma. She would have also noted its usual dosage range and rapid onset of action.

The nurse also erred by miscalculating the dose. This error reduced the overdose, of course. But if she *had* calculated the correct amount of 50 ml, she probably would have questioned such a large volume—and so discovered the doctor's error. To prevent such an error from happening to you, always look up an unfamiliar drug before administering it.

CONCENTRATION AVAILABLE				
Dose	1:1,000	1:2,000	1:5,000	1:10,000
0.2 mg	0.2 ml	0.4 ml	1 ml	2 ml
0.25 mg	0.25 ml	0.5 ml	1.25 ml	2.5 ml
0.5 mg	0.5 ml	1 ml	2.5 ml	5 ml
1 mg	1 ml	2 ml	5 ml	10 ml

Notes:

Error
Number

28

Not questioning a dose greater than 25 units of regular insulin for a patient who isn't hyperglycemic

A 56-year-old diabetic woman was hospitalized for treatment of foot ulcers. During her admission interview, she stated that she took NPH insulin: 70 units at breakfast and 30 units at dinner.

The morning after admission, the patient's breakfast and insulin were ordered held until some X-rays were taken. When she returned to her room, her doctor wrote the following order:

give her regular insuler 70 units subcut now

The nurse immediately administered 70 units of regular insulin to the patient, who then ate her breakfast.

A short time later, the patient said she felt dizzy. Her nurse called in the doctor, who asked about the dose administered. When the nurse told him she'd given the ordered amount of 70 units of regular insulin, the doctor realized what had happened. He'd meant for the patient to have her *usual* insulin dose, 70 units of *NPH* insulin.

The patient was immediately given orange juice, and she recovered from the insulin error without any further reactions.

Of course, the main cause of this error was the doctor's misleading order. But the nurse should have questioned a dose of 70 units of regular insulin for a patient who wasn't hyperglycemic. In fact, with the purified and human insulins available today, any time more than 25 units of regular insulin is needed for a single dose, the order should be questioned.

Medication errors with insulin are among the most common because insulin isn't ordered on a regular schedule as other drugs are. So be extra cautious:
- Make sure the patient has diabetes.
- Affirm that the dose and type of insulin make sense for each patient.
- Check the animal source (beef, pork, mixed species, or human) to ensure you have the one that's ordered.
- Have another registered nurse check each dose you prepare.
- Consider having the hospital pharmacy prepare certain doses of insulin. With this system, the pharmacist can check the accuracy of the order before he draws it up. Then he can label the syringe with the type of insulin, amount, and patient's name.

Mixing Dilantin with dextrose solutions

A patient recovering from a craniotomy needed phenytoin (Dilantin) to prevent seizures. The patient's nurse, preparing to administer the 9 a.m. dose of Dilantin, checked the doctor's order. The order stated that the dose could be given either through the patient's nasogastric (NG) tube or intravenously.

Because the NG tube had become clogged earlier, the nurse decided to give the dose intravenously. She attached a volume-control set to a bottle of 5% dextrose in water, filled the set with 50 ml, and added the Dilantin. She started the infusion and continued on her medication rounds.

Just a few minutes later, she heard the alarm from the infusion controller sounding in the patient's room. When she returned to the room and checked the I.V., she saw that the line had stopped infusing. She flushed it with saline and left again to administer the rest of her medications.

She was barely out of the patient's room when she heard the alarm sound again. This time she checked the I.V. line very carefully...and was horrified to see crystals forming along the entire length of the tubing.

The nurse immediately stopped the infusion and called the pharmacist. He told her Dilantin and dextrose were incompatible and that mixing them caused the crystallization. He explained that Dilantin should be given by a slow I.V. push.

The nurse checked with the doctor, who okayed the I.V. push. The patient suffered no ill effects from the incident.

The nurse could have prevented this error by reading the package insert for Dilantin, which warns against mixing the drug with *any* I.V. solutions. The insert recommends only a slow I.V. push of 25 to 50 mg/minute. In fact, recent studies recommend no more than 40 mg/minute.

In many hospitals, a large dose (up to 1 gram) of Dilantin is diluted in normal saline solution before it's administered. But this method isn't officially recommended. Whatever you do, though, *don't* mix Dilantin with dextrose solution.

Notes:

_____

_____

_____

_____

_____

Error
Number

30

Confusing "Inderal" and "Enduronyl"

A patient complaining of chest pain, weakness, and dizziness was admitted to a hospital emergency department. The admitting nurse contacted the patient's doctor and took his telephone orders, including an order for what she heard as "Inderal Forte," one tablet daily.

The nurse called the pharmacy to request the antiarrhythmic Inderal (propranolol), and when it was delivered, she immediately took it to the patient. Before allowing her to administer it, though, the patient asked the nurse to tell him the drug's name and explain its purpose.

When the patient's doctor arrived, the patient asked why he'd been given Inderal, which wasn't one of his usual medications. Puzzled, the doctor asked the nurse why she hadn't given what he'd ordered: Enduronyl Forte, which combines methyclothiazide, a thiazide diuretic, and deserpidine, an antihypertensive.

The nurse then realized she had misunderstood the doctor when she took his phone order, hearing "Inderal" for "Enduronyl." Giving Inderal had made sense to her since it *is* used for certain forms of chest pain. She assumed that "Forte" indicated an enhanced dosage form. Fortunately, the one dose of Inderal didn't harm the patient.

This error occurred because the hospital's system of checks and balances wasn't followed. The nurse didn't repeat the drug's name when she took the doctor's phone order. The pharmacist also didn't repeat the drug's name when the nurse phoned in her request. He thought that she'd asked for Inderal *forty,* that is, a 40-mg tablet. Although the pharmacist thought 40 mg of Inderal daily was an unusual order, he didn't ask the nurse to check back with the doctor.

To prevent such an error, follow these guidelines: Always repeat an order you take over the phone. If the drug being ordered doesn't sound familiar, ask that the name be spelled out. Be sure the doctor signs the verbal order within 24 hours, or according to hospital policy.

Know the drugs you administer. Don't assume an unfamiliar-sounding name is a new drug or dosage form. If necessary, ask the patient or his family what drugs he usually takes. If the patient has the drugs with him, ask to see them.

Finally, tell the patient what you're giving him and listen to his concerns. In this case, the patient discovered the error because *he* questioned a drug unfamiliar to him.

Mistaking "quinine" for "quinidine"

A young man who had a ruptured lumbar disk was admitted for a laminectomy. Because he had leg cramps, his doctor ordered quinine sulfate, 325 mg, to be given orally three times a day.

Five days after his admission, the patient underwent the laminectomy. During surgery, he developed premature ventricular contractions. The patient, who had no history of cardiac problems, was taken to the intensive care unit (ICU) after surgery so his heart function could be closely monitored.

In trying to understand what had happened to the patient, the ICU nurse reviewed his medication administration record. She discovered that instead of transcribing *quinine* sulfate, the ward clerk had mistakenly written *quinidine* sulfate. The patient had received this cardiac depressant for 5 days.

If the ward clerk's work had been checked more carefully, this error probably wouldn't have happened. But even if the transcription error had slipped through, the nurses administering the drug should have asked themselves why a patient with no history of cardiac problems was receiving a cardiac depressant.

To prevent this type of error, alert co-workers to drugs with similar names. Double-check transcriptions of drug orders. Ask yourself *why* a patient is being given a particular drug. If the order doesn't make sense, clarify it with the doctor.

Finally, except for malaria, quinine has not been proven effective for other indications. Perhaps it doesn't ever need to be in your hospital. Then it can't be mixed up.

Notes:

_____

_____

_____

_____

_____

Error
Number

32

Neglecting to document all medication orders in one place

A nurse was administering medications to a patient when he looked at the label on the unit-dose package she was opening. The label read *aspirin, 650 mg*. He told the nurse, "My doctor said not to take aspirin while I'm on Coumadin."

Surprised, the nurse wondered why she hadn't seen an order for Coumadin (warfarin sodium) on the patient's medication administration record (MAR). She knew if she had, she'd have questioned giving aspirin with this anticoagulant because aspirin increases the risk of bleeding and has an ulcerogenic effect.

The nurse checked the patient's MAR again but saw no order for Coumadin. She then checked his chart and realized what had happened.

In the chart was a special drug administration record listing drug orders written on a day-to-day basis. This record documented that Coumadin had been given daily for the past 5 days. But because this special record was kept with the chart rather than the MAR, the nurses who'd been giving aspirin to this patient for the past 5 days hadn't seen it. And the patient had been too ill during that time to notice what drugs he was being given.

The nurse alerted the doctor, who discontinued the aspirin. The patient's prothrombin time remained within a normal range.

This type of error could easily have been prevented. Special drug administration records, which are usually reserved for anticoagulants and cardiac medications that must be reordered daily, *are* useful because they provide extra space for recording monitoring variables such as pulses or laboratory test results. But when these special records are kept in the patient's chart, his MAR doesn't give a complete picture of his drug therapy. Therefore, if these records are used, they should be kept with the patient's MAR. When *all* medications are documented in one place, you can quickly check to see if any are incompatible.

If the hospital where you work has a system similar to the one that caused this error, try to get it changed so all medications are documented in the patient's MAR. And be sure to tell the patient what drugs you're giving him. (Note that the person who discovered the error was the patient himself.) He should be the final check in the hospital's system for preventing medication errors.

Not ensuring the dose makes sense for the patient

A 1-month-old premature infant weighing only about 5 pounds (2.2 kg) was hospitalized with an infection. Her doctor wrote the following orders for abdominal X-ray and abdominal girth measurement, as well as an order for ampicillin, 60 mg, to be given intravenously every 6 hours:

Because the loop of the "q" in the line above the ampicillin order looked like a "0," the ward clerk misinterpreted the order as *600* mg, which is what she transcribed on the medication administration record. The infant received three doses of 600 mg of ampicillin before a nurse questioned the high dose the following day. Although the infant suffered no ill effects from the overdose, she probably would have eventually.

Preventing this type of error involves more than writing orders clearly. Here, a pharmacist and three nurses, including the one who checked the transcription, had failed to question a daily dose of 2,400 mg of ampicillin for a 5-pound infant.

The lesson is clear: Know the dosage ranges of drugs you commonly administer. And check transcriptions carefully to ensure they make sense. Such diligence may save a patient's life.

Notes:

Error
Number

34

Mistaking the dram symbol for "oz"

A doctor wrote this order for a patient who had spastic colon:

During medication rounds, the patient's nurse mistook the dram symbol for "oz" and gave the patient 30 ml of Donnatal Elixir—a combination of belladonna alkaloids and phenobarbital. This was about six times the usual dose.

When the patient developed an anticholinergic reaction, the nurse checked the order with the doctor and discovered her mistake. Luckily, the patient wasn't harmed by the overdose.

As this error illustrates, apothecary symbols are frequently misinterpreted or used incorrectly. Because using these symbols can lead to errors, hospitals have all but eliminated apothecary symbols in orders. If a doctor prefers to write orders with apothecary symbols, the hospital should convince the doctor that using metric measures prevents confusion...and errors.

Notes:

Altering a pharmacy-prepared drug dose without first checking with the pharmacist

A patient suffering from acute asthma was receiving I.V. aminophylline. The doctor's order was for 375 mg per liter of fluid over 8 hours, three times daily.

After a few days, a nurse on the night shift noticed that the solution dispensed by the pharmacy was labeled *250 mg* of aminophylline per liter. She double-checked the doctor's order; it still called for 375 mg. Assuming that the pharmacist had mistakenly put only 250 mg of aminophylline in the I.V. bag, the nurse decided to correct the dose by injecting an additional 125 mg. She then administered the solution.

Not wanting to wake the pharmacist in the middle of the night to tell him what she'd done, the nurse left a note in the pharmacy mailbox describing the error and her action. When the pharmacist received the note the next morning, he immediately called the nursing unit. He *had* made a mistake. But the mistake was in labeling, not in preparing the solution. He had put the correct amount (375 mg) of aminophylline in the I.V. bag...but had incorrectly labeled it as 250 mg.

Because the nurse had added 125 mg to the bag, the patient actually received 500 mg of aminophylline. This one-time overdose didn't harm him, but if the error had been repeated, he might have developed theophylline toxicity.

The nurse, who was quite upset by the error, felt she had learned a valuable lesson: Never alter a pharmacy-prepared drug dose without first checking with the pharmacist. If he made an error, he should be questioned about it immediately, even in the middle of the night.

By the way, for the most part, hospitals today use a standard concentration of aminophylline or theophylline that avoids the unusual one ordered here.

Notes:

Error
Number

36

Not looking for the protocol after seeing an order for a diagnostic procedure

An inexperienced graduate nurse was asked to administer medications one evening. Although nervous, she completed the task without problems. When she arrived at work the next day, though, she was asked to fill out two incident reports for failing to administer certain medications to two patients.

What had happened? During her shift, the nurse had noted two new orders for gallbladder series the next morning. But she didn't know these orders initiated a well-established protocol that included administering Bilopaque capsules, which contain a contrast medium used in cholecystography. The nurse had no idea she was to administer these capsules the night before the test.

Because the capsules hadn't been administered, the patients' tests had to be postponed. The patients experienced added anxiety as well as a longer and more costly hospital stay.

Protocols often include administration of laxatives, sedatives, and contrast media. But unless the complete protocol appears somewhere in the patient's chart, parts of it may be missed, especially when a nurse is unfamiliar with practices on the unit. To ensure that this doesn't happen, preprinted orders should be placed in the chart.

To avoid making a similar error, be sure to look for the protocol whenever you see an order for a diagnostic procedure. If the protocol isn't there, check with the doctor or a nurse who's familiar with the unit's procedures.

Notes:
_____
_____
_____
_____
_____

Failing to give the patient or family members specific instructions for administering medications

A home health nurse was assigned to care for an elderly man who had a urinary tract disorder. He had just received an indwelling catheter, which needed twice-daily irrigations.

The man's wife volunteered to learn the irrigation procedure. The nurse showed her how to do it, using her own equipment and solution. Then she called a local pharmacy and asked them to deliver irrigating equipment and solution to the home.

The pharmacy delivered the equipment and solution, with several other containers of oral medications for the patient. The patient's wife carefully read the instructions on each container and followed them to the letter. One bottle was labeled: *Acetic acid solution. Use ½ cup twice daily.* So she measured exactly ½ cup into a glass and gave it to the patient to drink.

The patient immediately spit out the solution and refused to take another sip. His wife reported this to the home health nurse, who realized what had happened and explained that this was the irrigating solution. She assured the patient and his wife that he'd be all right because he hadn't actually drunk any solution.

An important lesson can be learned from this incident. Patients or family members should be given *specific* instructions for administering medications and performing procedures. This won't take any extra time, but it may prevent a serious error.

Notes:

_____

_____

_____

_____

Error
Number

38

Not clarifying an order that calls for "needing a B_{12}"

On a busy surgical unit, a doctor stated to a nurse that his patient "needed a B_{12}." Then he asked to see the patient's old chart. The nurse retrieved the chart from a file and started to ask the doctor about his order but was called to the phone.

When the nurse finished the phone call and returned, she found the doctor had gone without leaving any written orders. She was unsure whether he wanted the patient to be given a vitamin B_{12} injection or have blood drawn to determine his B_{12} level. She paged the doctor but got no answer. She decided that since the doctor hadn't mentioned a dose, he must have wanted a B_{12} level, so she wrote the order for it.

A few days later, the doctor stopped by to tell the nurse his patient had "gotten a B_{12} level" instead of a vitamin B_{12} injection. Because of the misunderstanding, the patient had undergone an unnecessary blood test and hadn't received medication he needed.

This error occurred because a rushed doctor didn't take time to write an order, and a busy nurse neglected to clarify his verbal order. Don't make the same mistake. No matter how busy you are, always clarify an ambiguous order before carrying it out. You'll be saving yourself time in the end...and you may be saving your patient from a serious medication error.

Notes:

Infusing concentrated potassium chloride

A nurse received an order to administer a liter of 5% dextrose in water to keep her patient's vein open. Soon after the nurse started the infusion, the patient's laboratory report arrived, showing she had severe hypokalemia. The doctor then ordered 40 mEq of potassium chloride to be added to the hanging I.V. bag. He also increased the administration rate.

The nurse drew the potassium chloride into a syringe and injected it into the solution bag through the additive port. Almost immediately after restarting the infusion, the patient began to scream with pain. The shocked nurse stopped the infusion and called the doctor. But by the time he arrived, the nurse realized what had happened.

After she added the potassium chloride to the bag, she didn't mix it with the dextrose solution. As a result, the concentrated drug flowed directly into the patient's vein, causing intense, burning pain. Fortunately, the patient escaped serious injury—probably because the nurse was able to stop the infusion so quickly. Transient hyperkalemia from an infusion of concentrated potassium chloride has caused death for some patients.

Many drugs that are added to infusing I.V.s can cause vein inflammation or drug toxicity if they're not mixed well. This problem occurs most often with nonrigid containers (plastic bags), since the area surrounding their additive ports tends to retain some of the drug.

To prevent the drug from pooling at the bottom of the bag, squeeze the drug from the additive port, then invert the bag several times to mix the solution. Using a needle of at least 1½ inches long to inject the drug, inject it over less than 5 seconds. Of course, you must mix well when using rigid containers (glass bottles), too.

Notes:

_____

_____

_____

_____

| Error Number | **Borrowing medications from a source other than the pharmacy** |

40

After delivering a healthy baby, a woman developed severe post-partum bleeding and was transferred from the obstetrics unit to the intensive care unit (ICU). Her doctor ordered several medications for her, including Parlodel (bromocriptine mesylate), 2.5 mg, b.i.d., which was to be given to prevent lactation.

The ICU didn't stock Parlodel, and because it was past 10 p.m., the pharmacy was closed. (Nowadays hospitals with 200 beds or more have 24-hour pharmacy service.) So an ICU nurse phoned the obstetrics unit and asked to have some Parlodel sent over so the dose could be given on time. An obstetrics nurse put four tablets into a medication cup, labeled the cup *Parlodel, 2.5 mg,* and took it to the ICU.

Believing the four tablets equaled 2.5 mg, the ICU nurse gave all four to the patient. Within minutes the patient developed severe nausea and vomiting, abdominal cramps, and dizziness. The nurse called her supervisor, who checked back over the sequence of events and discovered that each tablet of Parlodel was 2.5 mg, so the patient had actually received 10 mg—an overdose of 7.5 mg.

The patient was monitored closely for hypotension. She recovered after spending a very uncomfortable night.

Any time a system of checks and balances is violated, errors are more likely to occur. In this case, the system was violated when the pharmacist was bypassed, the drug was borrowed from a source not responsible for dispensing medications, and the medication cup was labeled ambiguously.

The error was compounded when the ICU nurse, who was used to the unit-dose system, assumed that the label described the cup's entire contents. She didn't look up Parlodel (a drug unfamiliar to most ICU nurses) in a drug reference or ask another nurse about its dosage range. Neither did she question giving more than two tablets for one dose, which is often a sign that the dose is not correct.

To avoid a similar series of errors, ensure that the hospital where you work has a backup system for obtaining medications when the pharmacy is closed. (You can help convince administration to institute this system by documenting the need for it.) For example, the pharmacist can set up a night supply closet stocked with unit-dose packages of commonly used drugs. If a drug is needed that's not in the emergency supply, a pharmacist should be called—to either suggest an alternative to the doctor or to come to the hospital to prepare it.

Until such a system is instituted, though, be extremely cautious if you must administer medications obtained from a source other than the pharmacy. Always look up unfamiliar drugs in a reference. Be sure to have someone else check the dose. And don't forget to double-check when you must give more than two units of the drug to complete a dose...a common sign that something may be amiss.

Notes:

Forgetting to add the drug to an admixture

A patient was brought to the recovery room after undergoing a carotid endarterectomy. Her arterial line showed a blood pressure of 190/100 and rising. So the recovery room doctor ordered a stat I.V. infusion of the potent antihypertensive sodium nitroprusside (Nipride).

The nurse, who was new to the recovery room, rushed to the medication area to prepare the admixture. She carefully reconstituted the Nipride and labeled the container of D_5W to show what she was adding to it. Then she brought the container back and gave it to the doctor, who started the infusion at a rate of 1 mcg/kg/minute.

The patient's blood pressure continued to rise. The doctor gradually increased the infusion rate to 10 mcg/kg/minute—but the blood pressure kept rising. The doctor checked the label to see if the nurse might have added the wrong amount of Nipride to the solution. But it stated the correct amount: 50 mg/250 ml D_5W.

Just as the patient's blood pressure reached 210/110, the I.V. container ran dry and the nurse went to prepare another admixture. To her horror, she discovered the syringe with the Nipride lying on the medication counter.

In her rush to prepare the first admixture, the nurse had forgotten to add the drug. She had reconstituted it in the syringe but then laid the syringe aside while she wrote out and applied the label to the container.

Flustered, the nurse ran back and told the doctor about her error. As she was doing so, another nurse quickly prepared the correct admixture and started the infusion at the original rate of 1 mcg/kg/minute. Within minutes, the patient's blood pressure started to drop.

Four lessons can be learned from this incident that will help prevent a similar error.

First and most important, always prepare an I.V. admixture *before* you label the container. Then check the emptied additive container to make sure you've added the correct drug and amount to the I.V. solution.

Second, don't let a crisis unnerve you or allow another staff member to rush you into cutting corners. Take time to pay close attention to what you're doing, especially if you have a lot of distractions.

Third, see that someone who's familiar with procedures is assigned to supervise an inexperienced nurse during a crisis. Remember, she's likely to be doubly nervous, have an incomplete knowledge base, and be more apt to make an error.

Finally, if you discover that you *have* made an error, report it immediately. If this nurse hadn't told the doctor of her error, he might have ordered the second Nipride infusion to be given at 10 mcg/kg/minute. This would undoubtedly have caused severe hypotension.

Notes:

_____

_____

_____

_____

Error
Number

42

Becoming complacent in using unit-dose Tubex cartridges and syringes

A patient was receiving intravenous antibiotics through a heparin lock every 6 hours. Every time a nurse administered an antibiotic dose, she had to follow standard procedure for flushing the lock and instilling 1 ml of 100 units/ml of heparin to maintain patency.

On the third day of this regimen, the evening nurse checked the unit-dose heparin Tubex cartridges in the patient's supply and was shocked to find they were all labeled *heparin sodium injection; 5,000 units/ml*. She realized that since one of these cartridges had been used earlier that day, the patient had received a heparin overdose.

The nurse notified the patient's doctor, who ordered a stat activated partial thromboplastin time study. The results were normal. The pharmacy was also notified and the heparin cartridges were exchanged for those of the correct strength.

Unit-dose Tubex cartridges and syringes go a long way in making drug administration safer and easier. But don't let their ease of use and similar appearance lure you into cutting corners. *Always* read the label before administering a drug: when obtaining it, when giving it, and when discarding the empty container.

Notes:

Not questioning an unusually high or low dose of insulin

A diabetic nursing home patient was hospitalized to control an infection that had caused her blood glucose level to fluctuate. When she returned to the nursing home, her doctor wrote the following order for a fasting blood sugar (FBS) test:

$$FBS \; \text{in a.m.}$$

Following standard practice at the nursing home, a nurse drew a blood sample and sent it to the laboratory that did the home's laboratory work. She then gave the patient her breakfast and usual medications, including insulin. She noticed that since hospitalization the insulin dose was higher than usual but gave it without questioning it.

Within a few hours, the patient began to show signs of insulin shock. At about the same time, the laboratory called the nursing home to report the FBS result. It was only 57 mg/dl, so the nurse gave the patient some sugar in orange juice. She then called the doctor to tell him the test result and the patient's condition, which by this time had improved.

The doctor explained that he had wanted the insulin to be held until he'd gotten the FBS test report. He had increased the dose when the patient was hospitalized and had intended to reduce it when she was transferred back to the nursing home.

This doctor was used to practicing in a hospital, where food and medications are routinely withheld until test results are available. He was unaware that most nursing homes send laboratory work to an outside laboratory, and therefore routinely *don't* withhold food and medication.

Both the doctor and the nursing home staff learned a valuable lesson from this error. The doctor learned that he must write orders more clearly. And the staff learned that unusually high or low doses should always be questioned.

Notes:

_____

_____

_____

_____

Making assumptions about what drugs the patient will be receiving

A nursing staff development director was asked to fill in as a staff nurse on the intensive care unit (ICU). Although she had worked in an ICU before taking the staff development position, the nurse felt a bit disoriented being back on the floor. So while the previous shift's charge nurse was giving report, the nurse glanced around the unit, checking the location of equipment and supplies.

After report, she assessed the condition of her assigned patient and looked briefly at his medication administration record (MAR). She read that he was receiving phenytoin for seizure control and was scheduled to receive what she thought was an intravenous dose of 60 mg of phenobarbital.

The nurse checked the patient's bin in the medication cart but didn't see any containers of phenobarbital. Assuming the pharmacist had forgotten to put the phenobarbital into the bin, the nurse signed out the correct dose from the unit's floor stock. She administered the drug as ordered and sat down to chart what she'd done.

When she looked at the MAR again, she was dismayed to read that the drug she was supposed to administer was *pentobarbital,* not phenobarbital. She immediately told the head nurse and the doctor what she'd done. They quickly checked the patient, then explained that because the two drugs have similar actions, he would not be adversely affected.

The nurse was still upset that she had misread the drug name. She also realized that if she'd listened more closely to the change-of-shift report, she'd have learned that her patient was being maintained in a pentobarbital coma—a measure used to control status epilepticus. The coma was to be maintained until the following morning.

Some basic guidelines can help you prevent similar errors:
• Listen to the change-of-shift report. You'll receive clarification of specific drug protocols that may not be spelled out on the MAR.
• Be sure to read the MAR closely. Don't assume that because you know the patient's diagnosis, you'll know what drugs he'll be receiving.
• Call the pharmacist if a drug scheduled for administration is not in the patient's drug storage bin. *Don't* go ahead and obtain the drug from floor stock. Doing so will violate the pharmacy's system of checks and balances.

• Most important, carefully check the name of the drug you're about to give, especially if its name looks or sounds similar to another drug name. Frequently, phenobarbital and pentobarbital are accidentally interchanged because their names look and sound alike and their indications are similar. Also, watch out for other drugs that have similar names and can easily be interchanged. There are thousands of possible combinations, like digoxin and digitoxin and quinine and quinidine.

Notes:
_____
_____
_____
_____

Error Number

45

Confusing "Colace" with "Tolinase"

A nurse in a doctor's office telephoned a neighborhood pharmacist to order a prescription for the stool softener Colace. The pharmacist filled the prescription and the patient picked it up.

Four days later, the patient called the doctor's office to say she'd stopped taking her medication because it had made her weak and dizzy. She'd looked up the drug name in a consumer's drug reference book, which stated that the drug was for diabetes. But her problem, she told the nurse, was constipation.

The nurse asked the patient to spell the name on the prescription label. It was Tolinase, an oral antidiabetic drug.

The nurse realized immediately what had happened. When she'd read *Colace* to the pharmacist, he'd heard it as *Tolinase*. The nurse explained the error to the patient and luckily she had no permanent adverse effects.

Ordering a prescription by telephone is a common practice, but not necessarily a safe one. Whenever possible, the order should be written and presented to the pharmacist in person. But if an order must be given by phone, these guidelines can help ensure that it's filled correctly:

• *Always* ask the pharmacist to read back the complete order to you, spelling the name of the drug and verifying the dosage.

• Write down the drug's name for the patient and pharmacist. Then, when the drug is picked up it can be checked. The original prescription slip would be best.

• Suggest that the patient buy a consumer guidebook to medications. Encourage him to look up the drugs prescribed for him before he takes them.

• Guide your patients to pharmacies where patient counseling occurs. Then, when the pharmacist says "here's your laxative Colace," the patient will have an immediate opportunity to correct an error since they would expect Tolinase for diabetes.

Notes:

Failing to read the label on a diluent container before preparing an injection

A 16-month-old girl was scheduled to receive 350 mg of cefazolin sodium (Ancef, Kefzol) every 8 hours to treat a pulmonary infection. To prepare the first dose, the nurse got a vial of cefazolin powder and a vial of diluent. She mixed the drug with 3.5 ml of diluent, then gave the 350-mg dose through the heparin lock.

The baby immediately went into cardiopulmonary arrest. The nurse called a code, and the baby was resuscitated.

After the baby was taken to intensive care, the nurse returned to the medication area. She picked up the used vial of diluent and was about to throw it out when she read the label. It said potassium chloride injection. Horrified, the nurse realized she had mistakenly used a vial of potassium chloride instead of the diluent she wanted, sodium chloride injection. The bolus of potassium chloride had caused the arrest.

This error could have been prevented if the nurse had read the diluent's label before preparing the injection. The rule you were taught in nursing school, to read a label three times (when obtaining a drug, when giving it, and when discarding the empty container), applies to diluents as well. Don't rely on appearance; in this case, for example, both sodium chloride and potassium are colorless and appear to have the same viscosity. Check the label: That's the only way to prevent such an error.

Notes:

_____

_____

_____

_____

_____

Confusing "Reg In" with "Reglan"

To prevent the nausea and vomiting associated with cancer chemotherapy, a doctor ordered 100 mg of I.V. metoclopramide (Reglan) for a patient who was to begin receiving cisplatin. The doctor wrote the order as follows:

Reg ln 100 am/100 NSS

The medication nurse, interpreting the order as "Reg In," administered 100 units of regular insulin to the patient. She thought the dose was unusually high, but because of an extremely busy schedule, she didn't question it.

When the nurse returned to the patient's room about 20 minutes later, she found him comatose. She called the doctor immediately and reported the patient's condition, adding that she'd given him the 100 units of regular insulin as ordered. The doctor answered that he'd ordered Reglan, not insulin, then instructed her to give the patient 1 mg of glucagon I.V. stat. The patient was given a second dose of glucagon about 25 minutes later and began to respond. He recovered within a few hours.

Several elements of bad practice led to this medication error. First, the order was carelessly written, causing it to be misinterpreted.

Second, the nurse didn't question the unclear handwriting. The dose was unusually high too. Any time you see a dose of regular insulin above 25 units, check it out to make sure it is correct. Today's purified animal and human species insulin don't usually warrant such a high dose.

To add to the possibility that these two drugs could be confused, metoclopramide is also indicated for diabetic patients suffering from delayed gastric emptying, which is caused by diabetic gastroparesis. Thus, a diabetic patient could conceivably have an order for either Reglan or regular insulin (or both). All the more reason to be alert for drug names that look alike.

Failing to keep patient care personnel up to date on new products

While a medication nurse was making rounds, she discovered that the transdermal nitroglycerin pad she had applied to a patient's upper arm an hour earlier was missing. She asked the patient about it, and he replied that "another nurse removed the pad when she gave me my bath."

The nurse quickly tracked down the nursing assistant who had given the patient his morning care. The assistant admitted she'd taken the pad off, thinking it was an adhesive bandage covering an intramuscular injection site. The nurse then explained that the pad was a form of medication, not a bandage, and was not to be removed except by a nurse or doctor.

You can avoid a similar error by making sure all personnel involved in direct patient care are kept up to date on the products and equipment they're likely to encounter. Good communication can prevent errors.

Notes:

Error
Number

49

Forgetting to check an unusual increase in a dosage of medication

A patient who'd been taking prednisone at home was hospitalized for surgery. Because the patient couldn't take anything by mouth after surgery, his doctor ordered hydrocortisone, 100 mg I.V. daily, to replace the oral prednisone. The patient received this for several days.

Later, when the doctor decided to restart the prednisone, he wrote the following order:

Prednisone 20 mg q 8 Hm

The unit secretary interpreted this order as *prednisone, 20 mg, every 8 hours* and transcribed it that way on the patient's medication administration record (MAR). The patient's nurse, who checked the transcribed order, interpreted the doctor's handwriting the same way and cosigned the transcription.

At 4 p.m., the evening medication nurse gave the patient the first scheduled dose of prednisone. When she charted on the MAR what she'd done, she noted that the patient had previously been receiving 100 mg of hydrocortisone daily. She knew that prednisone was about four times more potent than hydrocortisone, so she thought it unusual that the prednisone dosage was being increased.

The nurse checked the doctor's original order. She interpreted it as *q 8 a.m.*—not *q 8 hr*—and called the doctor to confirm her interpretation. Yes, the doctor said, he wanted the prednisone to be given once daily, at 8 a.m.

This patient was fortunate that the medication nurse caught the erroneous transcription when she did. Otherwise, he could have received an overdose of prednisone indefinitely, leading to immunosuppression.

Of course, the error could have been prevented if the doctor hadn't used the abbreviation *q 8 a.m.* to mean *8 a.m. daily*. Even so, the error still could have been caught if the patient's nurse had noticed the unusual increase in dosage when she was checking the transcription.

To prevent a similar error from happening on the unit where you work, check carefully whenever you see an abbreviation for *daily*. Such abbreviations have led to a variety of errors.

For example, the abbreviation *OD* (for *once daily*) has been misinterpreted to mean *right eye*. The abbreviation *q.d.* has been misinterpreted as *q.i.d.* when the first period was seen as an *i*. When *q hs* has been used to mean *every day, at bedtime,* it's been misinterpreted as *q hr—every hour*.

Besides double-checking the order when you see one of these abbreviations, always write out the word *daily* yourself. Finally, be sure to confirm any radically increased, decreased, or otherwise altered dosages when transcribing or checking medication orders.

Notes:

_____

_____

_____

_____

_____

Error
Number

50

Not being well informed about cancer drugs and their dosages

An oncologist wrote the following order for an elderly man who had terminal cancer:

CCNU 160mg PO, hs after dinner

After writing the order, the oncologist left the hospital and went on vacation.

The unit secretary transcribed the order on the patient's medication administration record. But instead of listing it in the "one time only" section, she mistakenly wrote it in the "scheduled medication" section. A nurse checked the transcription and signed it off as correct.

Ten days later, the oncologist returned from vacation. While reviewing the patient's chart, the oncologist discovered that the patient had received *10* doses of CCNU (lomustine), a potent antineoplastic drug, instead of the one dose he was supposed to receive. The doctor found that the patient had developed bone marrow suppression.

Since nothing could be done to reverse the effects of the overdose, the patient died a week later of kidney failure.

Why did this error occur? Unfortunately, each health care professional who had a chance to correct the erroneously transcribed order failed to do so. Two pharmacists were responsible for filling the order. Even though they discussed the dosage, they didn't check it in a drug reference.

Three nurses administered the drug, but only one checked the dosage in a drug reference. Unfortunately, this nurse misread the manufacturer's recommendation to "give every 6 weeks." She thought it read "give *for* 6 weeks." No one checked the oncologist's progress notes, which did state his intentions for this patient: "Will try a dose of CCNU."

Because most cancer drugs are toxic, even in therapeutic doses, overdoses can be especially harmful to the patient. Therefore, all health care professionals must use particular caution when administering these drugs.

Many hospitals are preventing such errors by confining cancer chemotherapy to a designated nursing unit. This gives the staff a chance to learn specifically about cancer drugs and dosages. Both an oncology nurse clinician and a clinical oncology pharmacist may be available to teach the staff, review drug orders, and answer questions.

Whether or not the hospital where you work has such a policy, make sure you're well informed about each cancer drug and its dosage before you administer it to a patient. Follow these guidelines for safe administration:
• Look up the drug in a drug reference.
• Check the patient's chart for the protocol or progress notes, which should further describe the therapy.
• Ask the doctor to go over his orders with you so there can be no room for misinterpretation.
• Have another nurse check the drug against the order before you administer it.
• Don't give the drug until you're satisfied you know how to give it correctly.

Notes:
_____
_____
_____
_____
_____

Confusing two patients with the same first name

Robert Brewer, age 5, was hospitalized for measles. Robert Brinson, also age 5, was admitted after he suffered a severe asthma attack. The boys were assigned to adjacent rooms on a small pediatric unit, and each boy had a nonproductive cough as a result of his condition.

During morning rounds, Robert Brewer's nurse took her patient's vital signs, then told his mother she had to get an expectorant the doctor had prescribed for his cough. When the nurse returned with the drug just 5 minutes later, the boy's mother told her Robert had already been given his medicine.

Puzzled, the nurse questioned Mrs. Brewer. She explained that another nurse had come in and asked her if the patient's name was Robert. When Mrs. Brewer answered yes, the nurse said she had the medicine for Robert's cough, and she gave it to him. Mrs. Brewer said she didn't know the name of the medicine, but added that the nurse had made Robert "breathe it in through a mask."

The nurse quickly went to the nurses' station to try to find out what had happened. There, she found a newly assigned nurse charting that she'd given Robert Brinson his prescribed mucolytic acetylcysteine (Mucomyst), which is administered with a nebulizer. Robert Brewer's nurse then realized that the other nurse, who was unfamiliar with the patients on the pediatric unit, had mistakenly given the mucolytic intended for Robert Brinson to Robert Brewer.

Both nurses went immediately to Robert Brewer's room and checked his condition. The mucolytic hadn't seemed to do any harm; in fact, it actually appeared to have improved his cough. But of course, any medication mix-up is potentially serious and a cause for concern.

This mix-up began when the newly assigned nurse obtained the prescribed Mucomyst for Robert Brinson. As she was walking down the hall, she realized she was unsure of his room number. But she spotted a young boy, so she entered the room and asked if he was Robert, adding that she had the medicine for his cough.

Unfortunately, the nurse had entered Robert Brewer's room. And because Mrs. Brewer knew her son was supposed to be given some cough medicine, she assumed that Robert's nurse had asked this nurse to give it to him.

This error could have been prevented if the newly assigned nurse had identified the patient correctly—by checking his identification band. Asking a patient (or family member) to confirm his name is not foolproof. A patient who is feverish, in severe pain, sedated, or preoccupied by his illness could easily misunderstand your question and give you inaccurate information. Similarly, a distraught family member may also respond inaccurately.

So always check the patient's identification band before giving medication, even if you think you know him by sight. That's the only way to confirm the first "right" of medication administration: the right patient.

Notes:

_____

_____

_____

_____

_____

Error Number	**Allowing interruptions to distract you when transcribing orders**
52	

A doctor telephoned the nurses' station and ordered 20 mg of hydralazine, intramuscularly, stat for a patient who had acutely elevated blood pressure. The nurse who answered the phone quickly jotted the order on a scratch pad.

While transcribing it to the doctor's order sheet, she was interrupted by another nurse, who asked, "Is the standard nitroprusside concentration 50 mg in 250 ml?" The nurse transcribing the order answered, "Yes, 50," and proceeded to write 50 mg instead of 20 mg on the hydralazine order.

The order was carried out by a third nurse, who obtained the hydralazine from floor stock and administered it to the patient. A short time later, a pharmacist reviewed a copy of the order. He immediately called the nurse who transcribed the order to tell her 50 mg seemed too high a dose. As he spoke, the nurse remembered that the dose should have been 20 mg and went to check on the patient.

The patient's systolic blood pressure had dropped to 90 mm Hg. The nurse alerted the doctor and continued checking vital signs every 15 minutes for several hours. The patient recovered without incident.

Interruptions are one of the leading causes of error. They're also a fact of life on most nursing units. Don't interrupt when you see someone else transcribing orders.

Notes: _____

_____

_____

_____

_____

Not calling the doctor and asking for the precise dose if he has ordered one tablet, capsule, or ampule of a drug

A doctor wrote the following order for an elderly, 95-pound (43-kg) patient who was unable to sleep:

chloral hydrate 1 cap hs

When the evening nurse went to get the drug from floor stock, she found only 500-mg capsules in the chloral hydrate drawer. Assuming this was the only strength available, the nurse signed out one capsule and administered it to the patient.

Later, the nurse began to wonder if chloral hydrate was available in different strengths. She checked a drug reference and, to her dismay, discovered that chloral hydrate was also available in 250-mg capsules. The nurse called the doctor, who said he'd thought chloral hydrate was available in only 250-mg capsules—which was the amount he wanted this patient to have. He asked the nurse to monitor the patient's blood pressure and respirations throughout the night. Then he came to the unit and re-wrote the order, specifying a dose of 250 mg.

Luckily, the one-time, 500-mg dose didn't harm the patient. But both doctor and nurse learned that medication orders must specify the exact dose. If you see an order for one tablet, capsule, or ampule of a drug, call the doctor and ask for the precise dose. Never carry out any order that's incomplete.

Notes: _____

_____

_____

_____

_____

Error Number

54

Confusing "Sinequan" with "Sumycin"

While a medication nurse was preparing for her morning rounds, she was interrupted by a doctor who was also making rounds. The doctor asked the nurse if she knew what was wrong with Mr. Stanislavsky, a 68-year-old man who was being treated for pneumonia. The doctor said the patient looked as if he'd suffered a stroke.

The nurse accompanied the doctor to Mr. Stanislavsky's room and found the patient unconscious. She took his vital signs: He had a slightly elevated pulse and low blood pressure.

The doctor immediately started an infusion of D_5W, first drawing a blood sample for a stat blood glucose test.

When another nurse came in to monitor the patient, the medication nurse left to review the patient's medication administration record and look for clues to his condition. She found that a new drug, an antidepressant, had been ordered the previous evening. The medication sheet listed the new medication as Sinequan (doxepin), 250 mg, every 6 hours. The nurse immediately recognized that this dosage was much too high. She also wondered why Sinequan had been ordered—she had not been told of any diagnosis of depression.

The nurse then checked the patient's chart and discovered what had happened. On the doctor's order form, she saw an order for the antibiotic *Sumycin* (tetracycline), 250 mg, every 6 hours. Apparently, the unit secretary had misread the doctor's handwriting, interpreting the drug name as Sinequan rather than Sumycin.

The night nurse, who had checked the orders transcribed by the unit secretary, didn't catch the erroneous transcription. And since the doctor had written the order in the evening and the hospital didn't have an evening pharmacist, it had been filled by a community pharmacist. Therefore, the order hadn't been reviewed by a hospital pharmacist, who would have been likely to notice the high dosage.

The patient recovered from the overdose, but he remained unconscious for a full day. Also, several laboratory tests were needed to monitor the patient's condition, adding to the expense of his hospitalization. Besides causing these effects, this medication error brought the patient's family additional stress.

This kind of error can be prevented by following a few basic rules:
● Before administering the first dose of a newly ordered medication, check the newly transcribed order against the doctor's order sheet.

• If you're unfamiliar with a drug, verify its dosage in a drug reference before giving it.
• Before giving any drug, ask yourself if the drug corresponds with the patient's diagnosis.

Finally, hospital administration can help prevent similar errors by establishing a 24-hour pharmacy service or enforcing a policy that the hospital pharmacist be contacted before any medication is obtained from a source other than the hospital pharmacy.

Notes:

Not being aware that using more than two units to complete a dose signals a problem

During a hectic day on an understaffed nursing unit, an inexperienced nurse was given the following order for a patient who had diabetic gastroparesis:

Reglan 10 mg IV stat

The nurse called the pharmacy for the dose, and a pharmacist arrived almost immediately with a bag containing five ampules.

The nurse quickly checked the pharmacist's label on the bag. It read: *metoclopramide (Reglan), 2 mg/ampule. 2 mg × 5 ampules = 10 mg. Use all 5 ampules.* She drew up and administered the contents of all five ampules by slow I.V. push.

Before discarding the empty ampules, the nurse checked the original label. She froze when she read *10 mg/2 ml*. Obviously the pharmacist had confused 2 ml with 2 mg. As a result, the nurse had given 50 mg of Reglan.

The patient was closely observed for the next 8 hours, but he developed no ill effects from the overdose.

This error could have been prevented if the pharmacist had read the manufacturer's label more carefully and the nurse had checked it before giving the drug. Also, she should have asked herself why she'd been given *five* ampules for one dose. Generally, using more than two units to complete a dose signals a problem.

When more than two ampules are needed for one I.V. dose, the drug is usually diluted. So giving five ampules I.V. push should have alerted the nurse that something was wrong.

To prevent a similar error: Do your own dose calculations. Scrutinize the manufacturer's label. Don't confuse ml and mg. And always check everything again when you need more than two of anything to complete a dose.

Notes:

Abbreviating "every other day" when transcribing medication orders

An elderly patient was receiving digoxin for congestive heart failure. When he developed kidney dysfunction, his digoxin dosage needed to be reduced. So his doctor wrote the following order:

digoxin 0.125 mg PO q o d

The unit secretary interpreted *q.o.d.* to mean once a day (q. = every; o.d. = once daily) and transcribed the order accordingly. The nurse who checked the transcription interpreted the order the same way and signed the transcription as correct.

The patient was given 0.125 mg of digoxin every day for 3 days until another nurse checked the transcription against the doctor's original order. She interpreted *q.o.d.* to mean every other day (q. = every; o. = other; d. = day) and called the doctor to check. The doctor confirmed that this was the dosing schedule he'd wanted. Luckily, the error was corrected before it harmed the patient.

This type of error can easily be prevented: Don't perpetuate the use of the abbreviation *q.o.d.* For one thing, it's frequently misunderstood, as illustrated by this example. For another, the *o* can be mistaken for an *i* when the order is handwritten, leading to an interpretation of *q.i.d.—four times a day.*

So always write out *every other day* when transcribing medication orders. And before using *any* abbreviation, ask yourself if it could be misinterpreted. When in doubt, spell it out.

Notes:
_____
_____
_____
_____
_____

Error
Number

57

Failing to take extra precautions when giving cancer drugs

An oncologist wrote an order for folinic acid, 10 mg, P.O., for a cancer patient who was receiving chemotherapy with the antimetabolite methotrexate. The order was written at night after the pharmacist had gone home, so the nursing supervisor had to obtain the drug.

The supervisor searched the pharmacy shelves for folinic acid, but could find only folic acid. Assuming the two drugs were the same, she sent 10 1-mg tablets of folic acid to the unit with instructions to administer all 10 tablets.

Because the patient's nurse wasn't familiar with folinic acid, she looked for it in a drug reference but couldn't find it. Assuming the supervisor must have already confirmed that folic acid and folinic acid were the same, she administered the folic acid.

The next morning when the pharmacist reviewed orders and drugs signed out during the night, he discovered the error. The patient suffered no adverse effects from the folic acid, but of course he didn't receive the benefits of folinic acid.

Folinic acid's proper chemical name is leucovorin calcium, which is why the nurse couldn't find folinic acid in the reference she checked. Leucovorin is frequently given after methotrexate administration to counteract some of this drug's adverse effects. This use is called rescue therapy, or leucovorin rescue.

To prevent such errors, cancer drugs should ideally be administered on oncology units staffed by personnel familiar with chemotherapy protocols. Practically, though, this may not be possible. But wherever cancer drugs are given, the staff must be taught *how* to give them...and have access to the protocols.

Also, hospital administration can help prevent cancer drug errors by establishing a policy that all orders for cancer drugs be reviewed by the pharmacist before the drugs are dispensed.

Finally, end the confusion between folic and folinic acid immediately by using only the proper name for folinic acid: leucovorin calcium.

Notes:

_____

_____

_____

_____

_____

Not keeping equipment out of children's reach

A 2-year-old boy being treated for pneumonia was receiving an infusion of $D_5/0.45NSS$. His nurse set the controls on the infusion pump for a rate of 40 ml/hour, then left the room.

When she returned 20 minutes later, the boy was playing with the pump's controls. Checking them, she saw that he'd changed the rate to 370 ml/hour. She quickly stopped the infusion and checked the amount of solution left in the I.V. bag. She calculated the boy had received 130 ml of solution in 20 minutes.

The excessive amount didn't harm the boy. But if drugs had been added to the solution, the increased rate could have had serious consequences.

This error serves as a reminder that patients themselves (adults as well as children) can inadvertently cause errors. So to prevent an error such as this, check an infusion frequently. Use an infusion pump only if it has an audible alarm and stops the infusion when the rate is changed. And when using an infusion pump with a child, be sure you place it out of his reach.

Notes:

Error
Number

59

Failing to clarify adjustments in I.V. flow rates

An elderly woman with asthma was being hydrated with I.V. D_5W. The flow rate was set at 125 ml/hour. She was also receiving a piggyback infusion of 800 mg of theophylline in 500 ml, set to flow at 25 ml/hour. When her doctor checked on her, he decided to increase the flow rate of the D_5W. He wrote on the chart:

Increase IV to 250ml/hr

The patient's nurse saw the order and increased the flow rate.

About 90 minutes later, the pharmacist received a request for a second container of theophylline. Puzzled, because the theophylline should have lasted 20 hours, the pharmacist called the nurse and asked what had happened to the first container. When the nurse said it was almost empty, the pharmacist replied that it should have lasted for several more hours. Suddenly, the nurse realized that the order to "increase I.V." meant the D_5W, not the theophylline.

The nurse stopped the theophylline infusion at once and assessed the patient, who by this time had started to vomit. She called the doctor, who ordered a stat theophylline blood level measurement and an electrocardiogram. The results of these tests indicated theophylline toxicity. The patient was given supportive treatment and recovered, but the error could have been fatal.

This error could have been prevented if the doctor had specified which infusion rate to increase. But the nurse shouldn't have implemented the order until she clarified what the doctor wanted.

Don't make the same mistake: When you receive an order to change a flow rate and more than one solution is infusing, clarify the order before adjusting the rate.

Notes:

_____

_____

_____

_____

_____

Not taking time to administer medications safely

60

A patient arrived at the clinic to get her weekly allergy injections. After waiting a few minutes, she complained to the nurse, "I always have to wait. Can't you hurry it up for once?"

Annoyed, the nurse grabbed a vial from the refrigerator, quickly checking the antigen's name on the label. She prepared the first injection and administered it. As she prepared the second, she glanced at the vial again and was dismayed to see another patient's name on the label. She'd given the wrong antigen.

The nurse quickly told the doctor what she'd done. By that time, the patient had begun to have trouble breathing. She was taken to a hospital emergency department for treatment, where, fortunately, she recovered from the allergic reaction.

This error could have been prevented if the nurse hadn't let the patient rush her, making her neglect to check the vial's label against the patient's chart. Because the nurse saw this patient every week, she thought she knew which antigen was hers.

The lesson: Always check a drug's label against the order, regardless of how well you think you know the patient or the drugs she's to get. Take time to administer medications safely.

Notes:

Error Number

61

Neglecting to put warning stickers on front of the patient's chart

A 7-year-old boy was admitted to a pediatric surgical unit to have an inguinal hernia repaired. When the nurse took the boy's history from his mother, she learned he was allergic to penicillin. The nurse noted this allergy on the boy's admission sheet, medication administration record, Kardex file, and her nurses' notes. She also placed an allergy alert sticker on the boy's bedside medication sheet. But she forgot to place one on the front of his chart at the nurses' station.

Later, a medical student examined the boy and also took his history. He knew the nurse had taken a history, so he checked the front of the patient chart at the desk to see if it had any warning stickers. Seeing none, he charted "no known allergies" on the patient's medical history. The intern and anesthesiologist, who also examined the patient, saw the student's note and consequently charted "no known allergies" on their respective evaluation sheets.

After surgery, the patient's doctor wrote an order for penicillin G, 1 million units, to be given intramuscularly. Seeing no warnings on front of the patient's chart, the recovery room nurse administered the penicillin.

Within a short time, the patient developed bronchospasm. He was given epinephrine and observed for several hours, then returned to the pediatric unit. No one on either unit related the bronchospasm to the penicillin.

The doctor then wrote a follow-up order for a dose of oral penicillin. The medication nurse checked the bedside medication sheet before giving the dose and was surprised to see the penicillin allergy warning. She notified the patient's doctor, who cancelled the penicillin order.

The nurse then put a warning sticker on the front of the patient's chart and told the rest of the staff what had happened. They realized that the bronchospasm must have been a reaction to the penicillin given in the recovery room.

The chain of events in this error began when the admitting nurse neglected to place a warning sticker on the front of the patient's chart. The medical student compounded the error by relying on the *absence* of such a sticker for his data on the patient's allergies. The recovery room nurse also relied on the absence of a warning sticker for her information.

Unfortunately, many people do rely on warning stickers (or lack of them) for allergy information. But these stickers were never meant to be the last word on a patient's allergies…the information *in* the chart is.

So to prevent such an error, always document allergy information in and on the patient's chart, following hospital policies and procedures. Before administering a drug, check for allergies in the chart, and ask the patient (or a family member) if he's allergic to any drug.

This last check is important when administering all drugs, but especially when you're giving penicillin, which causes more allergic reactions than any other medication.

Notes:

_____

_____

_____

_____

_____

Error
Number

62

Failing to send the MAR with the patient when he leaves the unit

A doctor ordered hydromorphone (Dilaudid), 2 mg subcutaneously, every 3 hours for a woman who had severe back pain from metastatic cancer. She was given an injection at 1 p.m., then an hour later was sent for her daily radiation treatment.

When she returned to her room at 3:50, she said she was in pain. Because her next dose of Dilaudid was scheduled for 4 p.m. and her vital signs were stable, her nurse gave the injection.

At 4:30, the patient's sister arrived to visit. Almost immediately, she called the nurse into the room, saying that her sister wouldn't respond. The nurse quickly checked the patient's vital signs and found her respiratory rate had dropped from 18 to 10 and her diastolic blood pressure had dropped by 15 mm Hg.

The nurse called the doctor, explained the situation, and added that the patient had last received Dilaudid at 4 p.m. But the doctor explained that the radiology nurse had called him at 3 p.m. to say the patient was in severe pain and couldn't withstand further treatment. So he'd ordered it given an hour early.

The doctor ordered 1 mg of naloxone (Narcan), which quickly counteracted Dilaudid's effects.

This error resulted from a combination of inadequate charting and lack of communication. Although the radiology nurse had documented the 3 p.m. dose in the nurses' notes, she couldn't write it in the patient's medication administration record (MAR) because this record wasn't in the chart. But she could have alerted the patient's nurses by calling the unit or placing a note on front of the chart. When the patient returned to her room, her nurse checked the MAR but didn't think to check the nurses' notes or doctor's order sheet before giving the 4 p.m. dose.

Send a patient's MAR with him when he goes to other areas for treatment or tests. And make it a habit to read the nurses' notes and progress notes when he returns.

Notes:

_____

_____

_____

_____

_____

Performing "routine" procedures routinely

Twice a week, an 81-year-old man who had end-stage renal disease came to a hospital to receive peritoneal dialysis. The dialysate solution was instilled, allowed to remain in his peritoneum for an hour, then was drained out.

While draining the solution after one of the treatments, the nurse noticed that a number of fibrin clots were blocking the drainage tubing. The standard procedure for this situation was to irrigate the tubing with a 20-ml bolus of a solution composed of 19 ml of sodium chloride and 1 ml of 1,000 units of heparin.

The nurse went to the medication room to prepare the bolus. Arranged on one shelf were all the additives needed for dialysate solutions, including 20 mEq/10 ml potassium chloride injection, 0.9% sodium chloride injection, and 1,000 units/ml heparin solution. She took some vials, prepared the bolus, and injected it into the patient's peritoneal catheter.

The patient immediately clutched his abdomen and cried out in pain. Startled, the nurse realized instantly that she'd used *potassium* chloride, which is extremely irritating to soft tissue.

She quickly called the patient's doctor, who ordered two rapid exchanges of dialysate to flush the peritoneal cavity. The patient didn't develop transient hyperkalemia or any other effect. But he did suffer intense pain for several minutes.

This error occurred because the nurse was so used to adding potassium chloride to dialysate solutions that she'd automatically reached for it when preparing the bolus. She didn't check the vial's label against a standing order.

The lesson: Don't perform routine procedures routinely. Check medication labels against standing orders. You may prevent a grievous error.

Notes:
_____
_____
_____
_____
_____

Error
Number

64

Not being alert for drugs with similar-sounding names

A woman in her second trimester of pregnancy developed premature contractions. Her doctor ordered ritodrine (Yutopar), which decreased them only slightly. So he then ordered progesterone vaginal suppositories. A new pharmacist received the order, obtained some suppositories, and sent them to the unit.

Later, the new pharmacist asked about the use of progesterone in premature labor and mentioned he'd just dispensed some called Prostin E_2. Alarmed, the senior pharmacist told him that Prostin E_2 is dinoprostone—a prostaglandin used to induce abortion. He quickly called the nursing unit and stopped the nurse from administering a suppository. She'd read the label but assumed Prostin E_2 was a brand name for progesterone.

Because progesterone and Prostin E_2 have similar names, are both hormones, and are both given intravaginally, they have the potential for being inadvertently interchanged. Obviously, this could have disastrous results.

To prevent such an error, stay alert for drugs with similar-sounding names. If you're unfamiliar with a drug or its name doesn't correspond with that on the medication order, look it up in a drug reference and call the pharmacist. Don't administer the drug until you're certain it's the right one.

Notes:

Neglecting to check both the pharmacist's label and the manufacturer's label

An unstable diabetic patient was hospitalized for debridement of a foot ulcer. Treatment included an infusion of clindamycin, 300 mg, in 100 ml of 0.9% sodium chloride solution every 6 hours.

The pharmacist prepared the solution in a piggyback I.V. bag and typed up a label stating the patient's name, bed and room number, name and strength of added antibiotic, and name of diluent. He placed this label over the manufacturer's label for the diluent and sent the bag to the nurses' station.

The nurse checked the information on the pharmacy label. Seeing that it corresponded with the order, she hung the bag and began the infusion. A few minutes later, the patient called her back to look at the portion of the manufacturer's label that was visible beneath the pharmacy label. The manufacturer's label identified the diluent as 5% dextrose in water, not 0.9% sodium chloride solution as stated on the pharmacy label.

The nurse quickly stopped the infusion and checked a drop of the solution on a reagent strip. Sure enough, the solution contained dextrose. The nurse notified the pharmacist, who prepared a new solution using the proper diluent.

Luckily, this patient knew enough about his disease and treatment to check both labels and discover the error. The small amount of dextrose he received didn't harm him, but a larger amount could have seriously compromised his condition.

Of course, most patients aren't that knowledgeable. To protect them from error, ask the pharmacist to leave the manufacturer's label uncovered when he adds the pharmacy label. Then be sure to read both labels when hanging an I.V. solution container.

Notes:

Error
Number

66

Mixing the contents of capsules with a food or medication

A patient receiving a liquid antacid containing magnesium and aluminum hydroxides (Maalox) developed a urinary tract infection. Her doctor ordered 500 mg of tetracycline every 6 hours.

The pharmacist dispensed a supply of 500-mg capsules of tetracyline to the unit. When the patient's nurse brought her the first capsule, the patient said she couldn't swallow capsules. So the nurse opened it, emptied the contents into 15 ml of Maalox, mixed the suspension, and gave it to the patient to drink.

The nurse administered several doses of tetracyline in this manner before another nurse stopped her. The second nurse explained that aluminum, magnesium, or calcium in any drug or food will chelate (bind) with tetracyline, preventing most of it from being absorbed. Because the tetracycline had been mixed with Maalox, the patient had received very little of it.

This type of error is easy to prevent. Whenever a patient can't swallow a solid oral dosage form, ask the pharmacist if an alternate form is available. Many drugs are available in liquid form or can be prepared as a suspension.

Notes:

Not completing medication administration and charting what you've done after preparing medication

67

A nurse on an oncology unit was preparing to flush a patient's heparin lock. A doctor came over to her, said he was going to perform a bone marrow biopsy on another patient, and told her to get the biopsy tray immediately. He told another nurse to prepare an injection of 3 mg of morphine.

The first nurse stopped what she was doing and got the tray. When she brought it to the patient's room, she saw the doctor administering an injection into the patient's I.V. line. He then proceeded with the biopsy. The second nurse came in just as he was finishing the procedure.

After they picked up the equipment and left the patient's room, the second nurse said to the doctor, "I guess you didn't want this after all." She showed him the syringe of morphine he'd told her to prepare. The doctor looked at the empty cartridge on the tray. He'd given the patient the heparin flush the first nurse had been preparing when he came to the unit. She'd set the syringe down when she went to get the biopsy tray, and the doctor had picked it up, thinking it was the morphine he'd ordered.

The patient wasn't harmed by the heparin, but he suffered unnecessary pain during the biopsy. Of course, the doctor was at fault for not reading the cartridge's label before administering the medication. But the first nurse should not have left a medication untended. The lesson: When you're preparing medication, finish administering it and chart what you've done before going on to the next task.

Notes: _____

_____

_____

_____

_____

Error
Number

68

Confusing "cyclosporine" with "Cyclospasmol"

A patient who'd just had a kidney transplant was transferred from the operating room to the intensive care unit (ICU). Her doctor ordered the immunosuppressive drug cyclosporine (Sandimmune) to be given orally according to the established protocol. The drug was dispensed and administered as ordered.

After 36 hours, the patient was transferred to the renal unit. Her medications were sent with her. When the renal nurse looked at the container labeled cyclosporine, she realized immediately something was wrong. Since she'd given the drug before, she knew it was available only as an I.V. injectable or an oral solution. This bottle contained tablets.

The nurse took the tablets to the pharmacist, who identified them as cyclandelate (Cyclospasmol) tablets, given to patients who have peripheral vascular disorders. She then called the patient's doctor and told him what had happened. He reordered the cyclosporine and told her to begin giving it immediately. Although the patient was at serious risk for organ rejection, the correct drug was given in time to prevent it.

This error was caused when a pharmacist confused the names cyclosporine and Cyclospasmol and dispensed the wrong drug. Because the ICU nurses were unfamiliar with cyclosporine, a fairly new drug, they didn't know its only oral form was liquid.

So be sure you know the drugs you administer. Before giving an unfamiliar drug, look it up in a drug reference. Remember: You're the last line of defense against medication.

Notes:

Misunderstanding a telephone order

A nurse took a telephone order for insulin, then transcribed exactly what she heard:

give 18 units NPH now and in 8 hours get a stat blood sugar

The patient, a newly diagnosed diabetic, was given 18 units of insulin immediately—and another 18 units 8 hours later (erroneously). A blood specimen was drawn when the first dose was given. The error was discovered when the patient questioned the second injection, and the nurse checked the order with the doctor.

Of course, the doctor had wanted the patient to receive *one* dose of insulin immediately, and a blood specimen drawn 8 hours later to assess the dose's effect. The extra dose didn't harm the patient, but he did have to be hospitalized another day so the doctor could determine his optimum insulin dose.

This error points out why telephone orders should be limited to emergencies. When you *do* have to take an order by telephone, though, be sure your transcription makes sense. To lessen the confusion in this instance, for example, the nurse taking the order could have specified a time for the blood specimen to be drawn. And she could—indeed *should*—have avoided the word *stat*. No wonder the blood specimen was drawn immediately.

The nurse implementing the order could have prevented the error by analyzing what she was doing. In this instance, drawing a blood specimen to measure glucose level when the first dose of insulin is given—then administering a second dose 8 hours later without drawing another specimen—makes no sense.

Don't take telephone orders if you can avoid it. But if you must take one, read the transcription back to the doctor first, then to yourself, to make sure it's perfectly clear. And if you must carry out a telephone order, be aware of its potential danger. Examine the order thoroughly before implementing it.

Administering a desiccant capsule

A new graduate nurse, preparing to administer medications, noticed that one of the doses on the cart was in the manufacturer's
original container. She carefully checked the label against the
medication order, then poured out the capsule—the last one in
the container. The capsule looked different from any she'd seen,
but she assumed it was all right since it came directly from the
manufacturer's container. She administered the capsule, then ordered a new supply for the next dose.

When the new supply arrived from the pharmacy, she noticed
the capsules were completely different from the one she'd administered. Puzzled, she asked the nurse manager about the discrepancy. When she explained that she'd administered the last
capsule in a manufacturer's container, the head nurse realized
what had happened. The new nurse had administered the capsule
containing desiccant, a drying substance that prevents medications from picking up moisture.

Luckily for this patient, the capsule passed through his body
without causing harm. Some patients have needed surgery to remove such capsules that wouldn't pass through their gastrointestinal tracts.

Most hospital pharmacists don't dispense medications in the
manufacturer's original container. But if the pharmacist at your
hospital does, ask him to remove desiccant capsules before send-
ing the container to the unit. If the container's kept tightly
closed, the medications probably won't pick up any moisture in
the short time they're stored on the unit.

And before you administer the last capsule in a manufacturer's
container, look at it closely. Most desiccant capsules bear the
printed warning: DO NOT EAT. Check it with the pharmacist if it
looks unusual and you're unsure. And if you're returning a manufacturer's container with only one capsule to the unit's drug supply, make sure that capsule isn't the desiccant capsule. You may
prevent a potentially serious medication error.

Notes:

_____

_____

_____

_____

_____

Mixing up medication cups

A night nurse was preparing medications for three patients when an elderly woman who had Parkinson's disease asked for some aspirin. After confirming that aspirin had been ordered p.r.n., the nurse poured two tablets into another medication cup, then picked up the four cups and started for the patient rooms. Recalling how the elderly woman frequently complained about getting her medications late, the nurse gave her the aspirin first.

As soon as the patient swallowed the tablets, the nurse realized she'd made a mistake. What she'd just given the patient was *not* two aspirin tablets but three *morphine sulfate* tablets meant for a patient who had cancer. She had mixed up the cups as she tried to carry all four at once.

The nurse notified the doctor and stayed with the patient while another nurse finished administering the medications and obtained a new dose of morphine for the cancer patient. Luckily, the elderly woman didn't develop respiratory depression or other adverse reactions to the narcotic.

Such an error is easily prevented: Never handle more than one patient's medications at the same time. And be sure to keep medications in their unit-dose package until you are at the patient's bedside.

Notes:

Error
Number

72

Failing to check patients' drug regimens for duplicate prescriptions

An elderly woman at an adult day-care center went to see the nurse for a routine checkup. The nurse asked if her doctor had prescribed any new drugs recently. The woman replied that she had "a lot of new pills" but couldn't remember their names. So the nurse asked her to bring them on the next visit.

A week later, the woman brought a bag filled with her current medications. After checking the labels, the nurse saw that the "new" drugs were simply generic formulations of brand name drugs the woman had already been taking. Because neither the doctor nor pharmacist had explained this to the woman, she'd been taking double doses of all her medications for over a week.

The nurse made an appointment for the woman to be examined by her doctor. She also alerted the woman's family and told them which drugs she should be taking. The doctor found the woman hadn't suffered any ill effects from the extra doses.

This potentially dangerous error could have been prevented if the doctor or pharmacist had told the woman that the "new" (generic) drugs were to replace the drugs she was already taking. Including medications with the directions would have helped. For example, *For blood pressure* may alert the patient if these are two drugs with the same purpose noted. Also, if permitted by law, the pharmacist could have labeled each container with both the generic and brand names.

Even if you're not a community health nurse, be alert for similar errors. During patient interviews, review the patient's drug regimen and check for duplicate prescriptions. Urge community pharmacists to put both the generic and brand names on a drug label. Finally, encourage patients to patronize pharmacists who keep patient prescription histories and review them when new prescriptions are ordered. This way, the pharmacist can alert the patient and doctor to any potential problems.

Notes:

_____

_____

_____

_____

_____

Not checking the five rights
of administration when comparing the drug with
the order in the MAR

A 75-year-old man recovering from a cerebrovascular accident was hospitalized for treatment of a foot ulcer. Four days after his admission, the medication nurse prepared to give him his bedtime dose of thioridazine (Mellaril), an antipsychotic.

The nurse obtained the dose from the patient's bin in the drug cart and compared it with the order in his medication administration record (MAR). The order called for 50 mg, but the dose she'd taken from the bin was labeled 150 mg. Checking the doctor's original order, she read:

The nurse immediately realized that though the unit secretary had transcribed the order correctly, the pharmacist had misinterpreted it, seeing the *l* on the end of *Mellaril* as the numeral *1* before the *50*. She called the pharmacist, who looked at his records and saw he had entered the order as 150 mg. He checked his copy of the original order and agreed he'd misinterpreted it.

The patient had received a threefold overdose of a major tranquilizer. Although he had become increasingly sedated, nobody had questioned why. Fortunately, he didn't develop more serious reactions to the drug.

This error occurred because the nurses giving the first three doses didn't check one of the five "rights" of drug administration—the right dose—when comparing the drug with the order in the MAR. Don't make the same error yourself. Every time you give a drug, know your rights: patient, drug, dose, time, and route.

Error
Number

74

Confusing "Seldane" with "Feldene"

A patient who had allergic rhinitis was given a prescription for Seldane (terfenadine), an antihistamine. A community pharmacist filled the prescription.

The patient took several doses but had no relief from his symptoms, so he called his doctor. When the doctor asked him what drug he was taking, the patient told him the name on the label was Feldene. The doctor realized immediately what had happened—the pharmacist had misread the order, giving the patient Feldene (piroxicam), an antiinflammatory drug prescribed for arthritis, instead of Seldane.

This kind of mix-up has happened many times. Because the two drug names sound and look so alike, they are easily confused. You can help prevent such mix-ups by remembering the differences between the two drugs. Seldane is prescribed for allergic rhinitis, comes in a 60-mg tablet, and is usually taken twice a day. Feldene is prescribed for arthritis, comes in a 20-mg capsule, and is taken once a day.

Ideally, a drug order should include its indication, strength, and dosage besides its name. As an extra precaution, verify the drug name by repeating or spelling it when taking or giving a verbal order.

Notes:
_____
_____
_____
_____
_____

Allowing a patient to leave the hospital before he has complete instructions for medications

A community health nurse visited a patient who'd just been discharged after having vascular surgery. The patient told her he was doing fine, but he didn't know how he was expected to swallow the two large capsules his doctor said he should take four times a day. He'd been able to get down only one.

The nurse asked to see the bottle containing these capsules. When she saw the label, she wasn't surprised the patient couldn't swallow them. The medication in the bottle was Neutra-Phos, a powdered phosphorus supplement packaged in capsules. The powder is meant to be emptied from the capsules and dissolved in a glass of water. But the label instructions said simply: "Take two capsules four times a day."

Apparently, the patient wasn't told how to take his medication. He was lucky he couldn't swallow more than one capsule because doing so could have caused severe gastric upset. The nurse showed him how to dissolve the powder, then called his doctor and pharmacist to tell them what had happened.

You can prevent such errors by encouraging doctors to write explicit administration directions on each prescription order, and encouraging pharmacists to type those directions on the drug label. Make sure the patient has received and understands the directions before he leaves your care.

Notes:

Error
Number

76

Preparing drug doses someplace other than the medication room or drug cart

A nurse in the intensive care unit was caring for a man recovering from a cerebrovascular accident. Because he'd developed cardiac complications, he was scheduled to receive 0.125 mg of digoxin through his central venous catheter.

The nurse obtained the digoxin and the heparin and saline solution cartridges needed to flush the catheter. The digoxin cartridge held 0.5 mg/2 ml, so she knew she'd have to discard 0.375 mg to get the prescribed dose. She couldn't find a syringe on the drug cart, so she decided to get one from the nurses' station and discard the excess drug in the patient's room.

The nurse went to the patient's bedside and flushed his catheter. After taking his apical pulse, she put what she thought was the digoxin cartridge in the syringe and began to discard the excess drug. Suddenly, she noticed that the label read *saline*—not digoxin. She picked up the empty cartridge she'd just used to flush the catheter. It was the digoxin cartridge.

The nurse quickly notified the doctor. The patient wasn't harmed by the digoxin overdose, but he did have to spend an extra day in intensive care for observation.

The best way to prevent such errors is by reading labels. A unit-dose system of drug administration will help since the exact drug dose you need will be prepackaged for you. If you work in an area of the hospital where this system isn't used, prepare syringes in the medication room or at the drug cart, not at the patient's beside. Reducing distractions will eliminate errors. And again, so will reading the label before administering a drug.

Notes:

_____

_____

_____

_____

_____

Not thinking carefully when calculating the dose of a liquid medication

A patient recovering from a total laryngectomy was scheduled to receive 20 mg of liquid morphine through her nasogastric (NG) tube every 3 hours p.r.n. A bottle of morphine containing a concentration of 20 mg/5 ml was kept in the medication room on the nursing unit.

During the evening shift, the patient told her nurse she was in severe pain. Almost 3 hours had passed since the last dose had been given, so the nurse obtained the bottle and measured the dose in a calibrated medication cup. Because the patient was so distressed, the nurse quickly administered the drug without checking the measurement.

As soon as she'd emptied the cup into the patient's NG tube, the nurse realized she'd made a mistake. Instead of pouring 20 *mg* (5 ml) of morphine into the cup, she had poured and administered 20 *ml*. She'd just given the patient 80 mg of morphine—four times the ordered dose.

The nurse called the patient's doctor, who ordered a naloxone (Narcan) injection to counteract the narcotic's effect. He also ordered charcoal slurries to be given through the NG tube. The nurse closely monitored the patient's respirations, blood pressure, and level of consciousness. Her respirations decreased, but she didn't lose consciousness.

These measures averted a serious reaction to the high dose of morphine. But the patient and her family were extremely upset by the error. The next day, to reassure the patient and provide a safeguard against future overdoses, the patient's nurse poured the correct dose of morphine into a medication cup and showed the dose to the patient. She told the patient to refuse any dose of morphine that appeared to be more than the dose in the cup.

This teaching turned out to be effective; a few days later, another nurse again mistakenly poured too much morphine from the bottle. When she showed the dose to the patient, the patient refused it.

The fact that this error was almost repeated illustrates why you must think carefully when calculating the dose of a liquid medication. Don't get so rushed or distracted that you confuse milligrams with milliliters. When you *know* you're distracted, have another nurse double-check the dose.

This incident also offers a second lesson: When possible, enlist the patient's aid in preventing errors. By teaching this patient how to check all of her doses, her nurses prevented a second overdose of morphine.

Error
Number

78

Preparing more than one I.V. admixture at a time

While making rounds, a doctor ordered an infusion of 100 mg of morphine in 500 ml of D_5W for a cancer patient in severe pain. He also ordered an infusion of 25,000 units of heparin in 500 ml of D_5W for a patient who had thrombophlebitis. Both infusions were to be started immediately.

The medication nurse, to save time, typed the two admixture labels first, then prepared the two solutions. She affixed the labels and handed the containers to another nurse, who then started both infusions.

An hour later, a nurse assessing the patient with thrombophlebitis discovered that his respirations were depressed. She called his doctor. After pulmonary embolism was ruled out, the nurse told the doctor that the patient had been fine before the infusion was started.

The doctor, suspecting a problem with the infusion, discontinued it and went to see the medication nurse. When he told her what had happened, she explained how she'd prepared a morphine and a heparin admixture at the same time. Since she knew she'd prepared the solutions correctly, she concluded she must have interchanged the labels.

That meant the patient with thrombophlebitis had been given the morphine infusion intended for the cancer patient, and the cancer patient had been given the heparin solution. The doctor ordered the cancer patient's infusion discontinued. Fortunately, the drug mix-up was discovered before either patient was harmed. New solutions were prepared and begun for both.

If your pharmacy doesn't prepare your I.V. drugs for you, resist the temptation to prepare more than one I.V. simultaneously. Instead, prepare one solution, then write and affix its label before preparing the next. This will ensure that you've labeled it correctly. Finally, investigate the use of manufacturer's premixed containers of heparin 25,000 units/500 ml and other drugs. These solutions are already premixed, well labeled, and reduce the chance of error.

Not questioning an unclear order for a drug available in different strengths

A 12-year-old child suffering from asthma was admitted to a pediatric unit. His doctor wrote several orders, including this one for sustained-release theophylline:

Theo dur 300 mg 1½ tablets b.i.d.

The nurse who reviewed the order knew that Theo-Dur is available in 200- and 300-mg tablets, so she wasn't sure how to interpret it: Did the doctor want her to administer 1½ 200-mg tablets to make a total dose of 300 mg, or did he want her to give 1½ 300-mg tablets, to make a total dose of 450 mg?

The nurse called the doctor at home and asked him to clarify his order. He said he wanted the patient to receive a dose of 300 mg. He didn't know a 300-mg tablet was available. So the nurse canceled the order and wrote a new one, which the doctor signed the next day.

By questioning an unclear order, this nurse prevented a potential overdose of theophylline. So whenever you see an ambiguous order, don't hesitate to question it. If you guess at the meaning, you may guess wrong. In medication administration, it's better to be safe than sorry.

Notes:

_____

_____

_____

_____

_____

Error
Number

80

Failing to clarify incomplete verbal orders

A patient who had rheumatoid arthritis came to the outpatient clinic for his weekly injection of Myochrysine (gold sodium thiomalate). The doctor examined the patient, then told the nurse to "give him 25 mg." The nurse gave the patient 25 mg of Myochrysine, as usual, and placed his chart aside, planning to document the dose later.

That afternoon, when the nurse was charting the day's events, she was dismayed to see the doctor had written an order for 25 mg of *methotrexate*, not Myochrysine. She immediately told the doctor what had happened. He explained that he'd changed the order to methotrexate because the patient's condition was no longer responding to Myochrysine. He assured the nurse that the Myochrysine wouldn't hurt the patient, but asked her to have him come back in for the correct medication.

The nurse called the patient, who returned to the clinic and was given the methotrexate.

In this instance, the patient wasn't harmed by the doctor's incomplete order. In a different situation, however, such an error could have serious consequences. So when you receive an incomplete verbal order, always clarify it (for example, "That's 25 mg of Myochrysine, correct?"). Also, wait to review the written order before giving a drug.

Notes:
_____
_____
_____
_____
_____

Forgetting to check transcriptions against original orders every 24 hours

A doctor wrote this order for a patient with a lower respiratory tract infection:

As he handed the multipart order form to the unit secretary, he said he wanted the first dose started at once.

The unit secretary immediately sent the pink copy of the order to the pharmacy and placed the yellow copy in a folder for the medication nurse. Then she transcribed the order onto the patient's medication administration record (MAR). When the medication nurse prepared to administer the first dose, she checked the MAR transcription against the yellow copy of the order, approved it, and started the infusion.

A few minutes later, the doctor returned and changed the order to 2 grams by writing a 2 over the numeral 1 on the original order form. No one saw him do this, and he didn't tell anyone about the change.

On the next shift, a nurse checked the doctor's order form against the patient's MAR and noted the discrepancy. She called the doctor, who explained that he'd changed the order but thought the change would have been noticed before the first dose was given. The nurse asked him to write a new order.

Luckily, the patient received only one incorrect dose because the nurse followed the routine procedure of checking all medication order transcriptions against the original orders every 24 hours. This is the best way to uncover any inconsistencies.

But doctors should be reminded to always write a complete new order (and notify a staff member) when they want to change one rather than alter an order already written.

<table>
<tr><td>

Error
Number

82

</td><td>

Not questioning insulin orders that don't specify the type of insulin

A doctor wrote the following order for an elderly insulin-dependent woman:

</td></tr>
</table>

Insulin 4o units daily
before breakfast

Since he didn't specify the type of insulin, the nurse assumed it was regular insulin and noted that on the patient's medication administration record.

The patient was given 40 units of regular insulin for 2 days. Before lunch on the second day, she developed signs of hypoglycemia. A stat blood glucose test revealed an abnormally low level of 40 mg/dl. She was immediately given a bolus of 50% dextrose injection, and her condition improved.

Both doctor and nurse were nonplussed by the patient's hypoglycemia. Trying to determine the cause, the nurse asked the doctor if he had increased the dose of regular insulin. The doctor replied, "Regular? I thought I ordered NPH."

The nurse then realized what had happened: When the doctor didn't specify the type of insulin on the order, she had assumed he wanted regular when, in fact, he wanted NPH. The patient's blood glucose level had dropped because she'd been given the fast-acting regular insulin instead of the slower-acting NPH. When the nurse explained what had happened, the doctor wrote a new order specifying NPH insulin.

To prevent similar errors, always question insulin orders that don't specify type of insulin. Also, as a rule of thumb, question any dose of regular insulin that's over 25 units. With the purified animal and human species insulins available today, such a dose would be unusually high unless the patient had severe hyperglycemia or ketoacidosis.

Interpreting the abbreviation "D/C" to mean "discontinue" rather than "discharge"

A patient with gastrointestinal bleeding had been hospitalized for over a week. On day 11, the patient's doctor reviewed his chart and decided he could be discharged the next day. In preparation for discharge, the doctor charted:

D/C meds:

Tagamet 300 mg PO q 6 h
Maalox 30 ml PO pc + hs
Keflex 250 mg PO q 6 h

A nurse interpreted this order as "discontinue the medications listed," and did so immediately.

The nurse discovered an error the next day when the doctor came to the unit and handed her three prescriptions, explaining they were for the patient's discharge medications. Confused, the nurse said, "I thought you discontinued all his meds." Pulling the doctor's order from the chart, she pointed to "D/C meds." The doctor explained that he used "D/C" in this order to mean "discharge."

This error illustrates how a little abbreviation can create a big problem. Usually, accompanying information will make the correct meaning obvious when an abbreviation has more than one meaning. Usually...but not always. To prevent such errors, be wary of any order in which "D/C" or other ambiguous abbreviations are used. And encourage doctors to double-check each order they write to make sure its meaning is clear.

Notes:

_____

_____

_____

_____

_____

Error
Number

84

Neglecting to check concentrations of medications ordered for children

An 8-year-old girl who had severe contractures from cerebral palsy was hospitalized for tendon-release surgery. The admitting nurse asked the girl's mother what medications she'd been taking at home. The mother said she gave her daughter one teaspoonful of Dilantin (phenytoin) suspension three times a day and one teaspoonful of phenobarbital twice a day.

The nurse relayed this information to the girl's doctor, who wrote orders for the medications to be continued in the hospital.

The girl was given 5 ml of phenytoin suspension before surgery and 100 mg of I.V. phenytoin during surgery. When she returned to the unit later that morning, she began receiving the maintenance regimen ordered by her doctor.

That afternoon, the girl started to vomit. Her nurse at first attributed this to the anesthetic administered during surgery. But when she was still vomiting the next day, the nurse became concerned and decided to investigate.

As soon as she checked the child's medications, the nurse realized what was causing the vomiting. The label on the bottle of phenytoin suspension read 125 mg/5 ml. The nurse then looked up the drug and found out that it was available in two concentrations—one for adults and one for children—and that the pediatric concentration was only 30 mg/5ml.

The nurse told the girl's doctor what she'd discovered. He immediately ordered a phenytoin blood level measurement and had the drug discontinued. The test results confirmed the nurse's suspicions: The girl's phenytoin level was 28 mg/liter—in the toxic range.

The girl's blood was tested daily until the concentration of phenytoin returned to a therapeutic level, at which time the maintenance regimen was resumed. Luckily, the girl developed no other toxic effects than the vomiting. But she did have to spend an additional 3 days in the hospital.

This error could have been avoided if:
• the admitting nurse had been more thorough in taking the girl's medication history.
• the doctor had verified which concentration of phenytoin the girl was taking and specified that in his order.
• the pharmacist had checked the girl's age on her patient identification card and had asked the doctor which concentration he wanted before filling the order.
• the nurse administering the phenytoin had looked it up in a drug reference book and been aware of its two concentrations.

Skimming over medication orders without checking for discrepancies

A doctor wrote an order for gentamicin, 80 mg, to be given intramuscularly every 12 hours to a 55-year-old woman hospitalized for pneumonia. The unit secretary transcribed the order as follows:

gentamicin 80 mg/IM q 12 h
(12 MN - 8 AM - 4 PM)

A medication nurse checked and approved the transcription without noticing the discrepancy between "every 12 hours" and the designated administration times, which are every 8 hours. For 5 days, the patient was given the antibiotic every 8 hours. On the fifth day, a nurse discovered the error and notified the patient's doctor. He ordered tests to determine the serum levels of gentamicin. As expected, they were in the toxic range.

The drug was discontinued immediately, and the patient's blood was monitored until the drug levels returned to normal. Thankfully, the error was caught before the patient developed nephrotoxicity or ototoxicity.

To prevent such an error, read medication order transcriptions in their entirety and check for discrepancies before administering a drug. Don't allow medication administration to become a mindless task.

Error
Number

85

Notes:

_____

_____

_____

_____

_____

Error
Number

86

Leaving the patient's room immediately after giving the first dose of an I.V. drug

A nurse was hospitalized for abdominal surgery. Because she had a history of mitral valve prolapse, her doctor ordered I.V. vancomycin and gentamicin preoperatively to prevent endocarditis.

The patient also had a history of drug allergies, so she was somewhat apprehensive when her nurse started the infusion and left the room. Within minutes, she became even more apprehensive, but she attributed this to her concern about the upcoming surgery. When she felt a hot flush on her face and neck, however, she thought she was having an allergic reaction.

She quickly shut off the infusion and called her nurse. By the time the nurse arrived, the patient's face and neck had swollen; her scalp itched; and her arms, chest, and thighs were red and covered with hives. The patient's nurse called the doctor, who ordered 50 mg of diphenhydramine, which relieved the symptoms almost immediately. Since the patient didn't develop any respiratory or cardiovascular reactions, the surgery was performed on schedule.

Any antibiotic, especially one that's administered I.V., has the potential for causing an allergic reaction. But vancomycin has been known to cause a severe rash (the "red neck syndrome") and prolonged hypotension, which is not an allergy but is related to the speed of the administration. Vancomycin I.V. must be given over *at least* 1 hour. Stay for at least 5 minutes with a patient who's receiving any I.V. antibiotic for the first time, and monitor her closely throughout the infusion. Even a patient who has no history of drug allergies may unexpectedly develop a reaction.

Notes:

_____

_____

_____

_____

_____

Using the proximal port of a pulmonary artery catheter to infuse drugs

A 55-year-old woman who'd just returned from coronary bypass surgery was receiving a slow infusion of I.V. dopamine to increase cardiac output. The drug was being infused through the proximal port of the pulmonary artery (PA) catheter because all other I.V. lines were being used.

When the nurse wanted to measure the patient's cardiac output, she disconnected the dopamine line from the proximal port, then injected the sterile solution into the lumen.

Suddenly, the patient's blood pressure skyrocketed. The nurse immediately realized what had happened. The rapid injection of the sterile solution had forced the dopamine remaining in the lumen into the patient's heart, elevating her blood pressure.

The nurse called the patient's doctor, who ordered the dopamine infusion discontinued. Fortunately, the bypass graft was not damaged by the rapid increase in pressure.

The lesson from this error is clear. Don't use the proximal port of a PA catheter to infuse drugs. As much as 1 ml of a drug could remain in the proximal lumen when you disconnect the tubing to measure cardiac output. Since this measurement requires a fast, forceful injection of up to 10 ml of solution, the drug in the lumen will be rapidly injected into the patient's heart. This can seriously injure him, especially when such potent drugs as dopamine, epinephrine, or nitroprusside are being infused.

In fact, infusing drugs directly into the heart through a central line is controversial. So reserve the proximal port of the PA catheter for its intended use: infusing I.V. fluids and monitoring central venous pressure. Whenever possible, infuse drugs through a peripheral vein.

Notes:

_____

_____

_____

_____

_____

Confusing "Delalutin" with "Dilantin"

A medication nurse, reviewing the medication administration record of a patient being treated for dysfunctional uterine bleeding, saw she was to give the patient an intramuscular injection of 125 mg of Delalutin (hydroxyprogesterone caproate). Since she was unfamiliar with the drug, she looked it up and verified that it was indicated for menstrual disorders.

When she looked in the patient's drug bin for the medication, however, she couldn't find it. Instead, she found a 250-mg ampule of Dilantin (phenytoin) injection. The nurse knew the patient didn't have a seizure disorder, and she knew of no other condition Dilantin would be indicated for.

She called the pharmacist and explained what she'd found. He then realized that he'd mistakenly read the order as Dilantin and dispensed the wrong drug. He immediately sent the proper dose of Delalutin to the unit and retrieved the Dilantin.

This nurse's diligence prevented a medication error. So be sure to follow her example in your own practice: Always check the patient's diagnosis, and look up drugs you're not familiar with before administering them. Don't give what's in a patient's drug bin just because it's there; compare the drugs with the order.

Notes:

Concentrating on more than one task at a time

The charge nurse on a busy medical/surgical unit was feeling rushed because she was also responsible for administering all the I.V. push medications. While she was making rounds, she was dismayed to see bright red urine in Mr. Gregario's collection bag. She alerted his doctor, reminding him that the patient was receiving heparin. The doctor ordered a stat activated partial thromboplastin time (APTT) test and told her to hold the heparin.

A short while later, when she was preparing to give the I.V. medications, the nurse noted that a dose of heparin was ordered for Mr. Simmons. She carefully prepared the dose, checked it against his medication administration record...then walked into Mr. Gregario's room and gave the heparin to him.

The nurse was horrified when she realized what she'd done. She called the doctor, who administered protamine sulfate to counteract the heparin's effect; he also ordered another APTT test. Luckily, Mr. Gregario was not harmed by the unordered heparin.

This incident illustrates how even the most careful nurse can make a mistake. In this instance, the busy nurse was so worried about Mr. Gregario and his hematuria—associating his problem with heparin—that she gave the heparin to him.

To prevent such an error, *always* check a patient's armband before giving him a drug. And even in a pressure-cooker situation, concentrate on one task at a time.

Notes: _____

_____

_____

_____

_____

Error
Number

90

Being careless when stocking drugs

After giving birth, a patient on the labor and delivery unit began to bleed heavily. The doctor ordered a stat dose of Ergotrate (ergonovine maleate) to stop the bleeding.

The nurse went to the unit's stock of emergency drugs and took an ampule from the bin that was labeled *Ergotate*. As she broke open the ampule, she read its label and was surprised to see it said *epinephrine*. She quickly discarded the ampule and obtained another one from the same bin, confirming first that it was labeled Ergotrate. She administered the correct drug, and the patient eventually stopped bleeding.

This kind of close call can happen on any unit. Many emergency drugs appear similar because they're packaged in ampules; furthermore, the ampule labels can be difficult to read. If the pharmacist accidentally sends two types of drugs in one bag and the nurse stocking them doesn't realize it, she could easily put both drugs into one bin.

There are several ways to prevent this type of error:
• When stocking ampules, read each one's label, even though the bag containing the ampules is labeled with one drug name. By the same token, read an ampule's label when you obtain it for administration, even though its bin is also labeled.
• Remind all nurses on the unit that ampules are easily misstocked. Place a note in each drug bin reminding co-workers to read the ampule labels.
• Talk to the hospital pharmacist about getting drugs in containers other than ampules. Single-dose vials, prefilled syringes, and premixed solutions are some alternatives.

Notes:
_____
_____
_____
_____
_____

Not verifying the concentration of liquid medications

A medication nurse was given this order for a patient with cancer pain:

morphine soln 7 ml q 3 h

The nurse took a bottle of liquid morphine from the narcotics supply, poured out 7 ml, and administered it. Three hours later, she repeated the dose.

An hour after the second dose was given, the patient was found unconscious and barely breathing. Her skin was cold, pale, and moist. Suspecting a morphine overdose, her doctor ordered naloxone (Narcan). Three 0.25-mg doses had to be given before the patient revived.

Both the doctor and nurse wondered how two 14-mg doses of morphine could affect the patient so severely. The nurse decided to look more closely at the bottle of morphine she had used to obtain the dose. She was shocked when she read the label. The concentration of morphine was not 2 mg/ml, as she had thought, but *20* mg/ml. She had given the patient 280 mg of morphine.

The patient was lucky that her condition was discovered and treated promptly; such a high dose of morphine could have been fatal. This error happened because the nurse left out a basic but crucial step in medication administration—reading the label. She didn't know two concentrations of liquid morphine were available and simply poured the amount of milliliters ordered.

To prevent such an error, encourage doctors to write orders for liquid medications in milligrams rather than milliliters. Ask pharmacists to clearly indicate the concentrations of these drugs on their labels. And of course, always verify that you have the correct concentration when obtaining a liquid medication.

Notes:

_____

_____

_____

_____

| Error Number **92** | **Preparing more than one medication at a time** |

A patient on a cardiac care unit was receiving a continuous infusion of 50 mg of Nipride (sodium nitroprusside), diluted in 250 ml of D_5W, to improve cardiac output. As the infusion was running out, the doctor ordered 40 mg of Lasix (furosemide, frusemide), I.V. push. The nurse obtained a 40-mg vial of Lasix and a 50-mg vial of Nipride. She reconstituted the Nipride in the vial, then set it down next to the Lasix to get a new bag of D_5W from the supply closet.

When the nurse returned, the doctor asked her to give the bolus of Lasix immediately. She picked up the vial, withdrew the drug, and injected it into the patient's I.V. line.

Suddenly, the patient's blood pressure dropped. The nurse called the doctor, then took a closer look at the vial she'd just used. It was the vial of Nipride.

Fortunately, the patient's I.V. had infiltrated, so she didn't get the full bolus of Nipride. After a vasopressor was administered, her blood pressure rose to a safe level.

This potentially fatal error occurred because the two vials were similar in size and color and because the nurse neglected to read the label when she withdrew what she thought was Lasix. Remember, *always* read labels when administering medications. Don't rely on the container's appearance. To further reduce the chance of error, prepare and administer only one medication at a time.

Notes:

_____

_____

_____

_____

_____

Combining Dilantin with dextrose

An 89-year-old former stroke patient was admitted with a diagnosis of myocardial infarction. When she developed seizures, her doctor ordered several medications, including Dilantin (phenytoin), 100 mg, slow I.V. push, every 8 hours.

The patient was already receiving an infusion of D_5W in her right hand. Because the patient's veins were so fragile, the nurse didn't want to start another I.V. So, knowing that combining Dilantin with dextrose can cause precipitation, she diluted the drug with 10 ml of saline injection. After flushing the running I.V. with normal saline solution, she slowly injected the Dilantin through the Y site, then flushed the line again.

An hour later, the nurse observed signs of severe phlebitis in the patient's right hand. She alerted the doctor, who ordered a continuous infusion of heparin at 1,000 units/hour. The hand was saved, but the patient had to be hospitalized for 10 days of heparin therapy.

This medication error shows just *how* incompatible Dilantin and dextrose are. Even though the nurse diluted the Dilantin and flushed the line with saline, a precipitate still formed. The patient's small veins and decreased peripheral circulation undoubtedly contributed to the severity of the reaction.

When administering I.V. Dilantin to a patient receiving D_5W, be careful not to repeat this nurse's mistake. The only way to prevent precipitation in this case is to inject the Dilantin directly into a large vein or into a running infusion of normal saline.

Notes:

Error
Number

94

Using unorthodox containers for medications

A 65-year-old man with thyroid cancer was admitted to a long-term care facility. Because the patient was having difficulty swallowing, the pharmacist dispensed the prescribed oral morphine solution in infection syringes with the needles removed.

The patient's nurses knew that morphine dispensed in this form was meant to be given orally. However, the registry nurse assigned to the patient one night was unaware of this. So when she saw the syringe containing the medication, with nothing on the label to indicate that it was an oral drug, she attached a needle and injected the morphine solution into the patient's buttock.

Later that night, the patient asked one of the staff nurses why he'd been given an injection. The nurse checked with the registry nurse and found out what had happened. She quickly alerted the pharmacist, who reassured her that the morphine would probably be absorbed systemically. But he warned that the injection could cause an abscess. (Fortunately, this didn't happen.)

As a result of this error, the staff nurses and pharmacist drew up the following guidelines, designed to prevent the use of unorthodox, improperly labeled containers for medications:
• Don't put oral drugs in syringes normally used for injection. Instead, use oral syringes, which can't accommodate a needle.
• Clearly label these syringes "For oral use only."
• Inform all temporary staff members about methods of medication administration. This information should be given during shift report and should be included on the patient's chart.

Notes:

_____

_____

_____

_____

_____

Giving unclear administration directions

A charge nurse on a medical/surgical unit discovered that a patient's blood pressure had risen to 200/150. She called the doctor, who ordered 10 mg of nifedipine (Procardia, Adalat), to be given sublingually. Relaying this order to the patient's nurse, a new employee, the charge nurse emphasized that the capsule must be given sublingually for the drug to work quickly.

A few minutes later, the charge nurse checked the patient and was greeted with the question: "How is this pill supposed to dissolve under my tongue?"

The charge nurse realized immediately that the new nurse had misunderstood her directions. Apparently, the new nurse didn't know that a sublingual form of nifedipine isn't available in the United States or Canada. However, the drug may be given sublingually by perforating the capsule about 10 times with a 25-gauge needle and squeezing its contents under the patient's tongue. This form of sublingual administration, which may be used only with oral nifedipine capsules, treats severe hypertension and vasospastic angina. After discarding the first capsule, the charge nurse administered another one in the proper manner. When she checked back a short while later, the patient's blood pressure had dropped to 160/110.

This kind of medication error is easily avoided. Just make sure you review and demonstrate unusual administration routes for staff members, especially new employees. The route should also be documented in the patient's chart.

Notes:

Error
Number

96

Forgetting to check the diluent concentration on the label

A patient hospitalized with deep vein thrombosis developed a pleural effusion. The surgeon performed a thoracentesis, draining 1,400 ml of blood-tinged fluid. He then wrote an order to resume the patient's heparin drip at the previous rate—1,000 units/hour.

The patient's nurse called in the order and the pharmacist sent a bag to the unit, already mixed and labeled. The nurse quickly hung the bag and set the correct infusion rate.

When the night nurse came on duty a few hours later, she was puzzled to see that the patient's I.V. bag contained 20,000 units of heparin in 500 ml of D_5W. She recalled that the concentration the night before had been 20,000 units in *1,000* ml.

She called the surgeon. He made it clear that he wanted the same concentration as before. Following his orders, the nurse obtained the correct concentration and started the infusion at a lower rate. The patient's partial thromboplastin time was high, as expected, but it dropped to a normal level within a few hours.

Three people contributed to this potentially fatal error. The surgeon failed to specify the concentration in his order. The pharmacist filled the order even though it was incomplete. And the nurse forgot to check the concentration on the label.

This error could have been prevented if these practitioners had been more careful. Better yet, if the hospital had established a standard concentration for heparin (and all critical care drug infusions), only the number of units per hour would have to be ordered. Such a practice is an excellent way to decrease errors.

Notes:

_____

_____

_____

_____

Not questioning duplication of doses

A patient discharged after a cholecystectomy developed a wound infection and had to be readmitted. His doctor ordered antibiotics for the infection, Demerol (meperidine) for severe pain, and Tylenol (acetaminophen) for less severe pain.

When the patient's condition improved and his pain decreased, the doctor discontinued the Demerol and ordered Tylenol with Codeine No. 2, two tablets q4h, in its place. He forgot that his original order for Tylenol, 325 mg, two tablets q4h, hadn't been discontinued.

The nurse who transcribed the Tylenol with Codeine No. 2 order didn't see the original order for Tylenol because it was on a separate medication sheet. So for 10 days the patient received two tablets of regular Tylenol *and* two tablets of Tylenol with Codeine No. 2 (which contains 300 mg of acetaminophen per tablet) every 4 hours—a daily dose of 7,500 mg of acetaminophen.

The patient's doctor discovered the error when routine laboratory tests showed elevated liver enzymes. Screening the patient's medication administration record (MAR) for a clue, he found the double doses. The doctor immediately discontinued both Tylenol orders and ordered the patient's liver function monitored daily. Luckily, the enzyme levels returned to normal within a week.

The doctor erred by not reviewing the patient's current medications when ordering the Tylenol with Codeine No. 2. But the patient's nurses bear some of the blame as well—not one questioned the duplication of doses.

To prevent such errors, review the patient's MAR whenever a new drug is ordered. And when administering drugs, keep alert for duplications.

Notes: _____

_____

_____

_____

Error
Number

98

Violating hospital protocol

A nurse was hospitalized for removal of a cyst. Her doctor ordered a preoperative infusion of cefazolin, 1 gram in 100 ml of D$_5$W. When the container was hung, the nurse-patient instinctively checked the label. She was surprised to see another patient's name on it, even though the drug and dose information was correct.

She told her nurse about the label. The nurse explained that although the label had someone else's name on it, the bag contained the drug prescribed for her. The pharmacist had prepared the infusion for another patient before learning that the order had been discontinued. He said it was okay to use it for the nurse-patient.

Not satisfied with this explanation, the nurse-patient protested to her doctor. On his order, a new infusion was prepared, labeled correctly, and hung.

This incident shows poor practice on the part of both the pharmacist and nurse. Any medication dispensed but not used should be returned to the pharmacy. If it can be used for another patient, it must be checked to see that it's been sealed and stored correctly, then relabeled.

Violating this protocol can easily lead to medication errors. Besides, common sense tells you that giving a patient a medication that has someone else's name on the label is no way to gain that patient's trust.

Notes:

Relying on memory rather than labeling syringes after preparing an injection

While assisting a surgeon during eye surgery, a nurse prepared injections of gentamicin and balanced salt solution but didn't bother to label either one. Gentamicin is injected under the conjunctiva to prevent postoperative infection; balanced salt solution is sometimes injected directly into the eye to restore intraocular pressure.

Toward the end of the operation, the surgeon asked for the balanced salt solution. The nurse handed him one of the two syringes and he injected its contents into the patient's eye. As he did so, the nurse realized that she had given him the syringe containing the gentamicin.

The mistake was irrevocable—and tragic. The patient became blind in that eye.

This unfortunate incident occurred because of a mistake that's easily avoided—failing to label syringes. The nurse apparently thought she would remember which syringe was which.

In most cases, of course, the pharmacist will prepare and label injections. This is routine practice in many hospitals, as is the dispensing of commercially available prefilled syringes.

But when you must prepare an injection, don't make the mistake just described. Always label the syringe immediately. (The pharmacist can supply typed labels to make this step even easier.) Keep the vial with the syringe, and show the vial to the doctor when he's ready to administer the drug.

Notes:

Error
Number

100

Administering medication I.V. when the MAR clearly states it should be given orally

A patient recovering from a total hip replacement developed an infection around the prosthesis. A 1-month course of antibiotics eventually brought the infection under control. Unfortunately, the antibiotics caused pseudomembranous colitis, a serious adverse reaction. The doctor ordered oral vancomycin (Vancocin), commonly used to treat this condition.

Although oral forms of vancomycin are available, the pharmacist had only injectable vancomycin in stock. Following the accepted procedure, he added water to the contents of an injectable vial so the drug could be given orally. But he neglected to specify the oral route on the vial's label.

When the medication nurse received the vial, she failed to check the patient's medication administration record (MAR), which clearly stated that the drug was to be given orally. She drew up the vial's contents and administered the medication I.V., through a volume-control set.

The patient suffered no harm from this error, but neither did he receive any benefit from the drug—I.V. vancomycin is relatively ineffective for pseudomembranous colitis. Both the pharmacist and nurse contributed to this error. The pharmacist dispensed an injectable drug without noting that it was to be given orally. The nurse gave the drug without first checking the MAR.

Don't make the same mistake: Always verify a drug's administration route. And remember that vancomycin should be given orally for pseudomembranous colitis.

Notes:

Mistaking a slash for the number 1

A nurse, following a doctor's written order, gave her diabetic patient 40 units of lente insulin with 120 units of regular insulin. A short while later, she realized the patient was showing signs of an insulin reaction. She called the pharmacist, told him what she'd administered, and asked him to check the original order. It looked like this:

The pharmacist interpreted the order as 40 units of lente insulin with *20* units of regular insulin. He realized at once what the nurse had done—she'd read the slash before the 20 as a "1." As a result, she'd given an insulin overdose.

The nurse alerted the patient's doctor, who ordered a stat blood glucose test. As suspected, the patient was hypoglycemic. Several doses of I.V. glucose were needed to bring her glucose level back to normal.

A doctor's shorthand—using a slash instead of writing out "with"—caused the nurse to misinterpret his order. Regrettably, she didn't stop to consider that 120 units of regular insulin was an unusually large dose.

Don't let medication administration become a mindless process. Think an order through before you carry it out. And watch for those slashes that could be mistaken for a "1."

Notes:

_____

_____

_____

_____

_____

Error
Number

102

Confusing the identity of two patients with the same last name

A standing order for temazepam had been written for "A. Lambert," a nursing home patient. One night a nursing assistant told the medication nurse that "Lambert" was asking for a sleeping pill. The nurse checked her list of patients for whom sleep medications had been ordered. Seeing an "A. Lambert" on the list, she went to Mrs. Lambert's room, checked her armband (which read "A. Lambert"), and administered the temazepam.

About 30 minutes later, the nursing assistant mentioned that *Mr*. Lambert was still asking for his sleeping pill. The medication nurse was quite surprised to learn there were *two* A. Lamberts on the unit—Alice Lambert and her husband Alan. She had given the temazepam to the wrong Lambert.

The mix-up caused no harm, but it does illustrate the unusual ways that drug administration errors can occur. To protect your patients from such errors, adopt these guidelines:
• If two patients with the same last name are admitted to your unit, inform staff members of this fact during report, and make a note on the charts.
• Make sure all patients' armbands list both first and last names.
• Use both first and last names when referring to patients.
• Before giving any medication, check the patient's medication administration record, not just a list of patients receiving a particular type of medication.

Notes:

_____

_____

_____

_____

_____

Interpreting the number "15" as "50"

A woman experiencing severe hypertension was admitted to an intensive care unit (ICU). Her doctor called in an order for 15 mg of hydralazine to be given intravenously every 2 hours. Because the doctor spoke with an accent, the nurse misunderstood him. She thought he said *50* mg.

After obtaining three 20-mg vials of hydralazine, the nurse drew up the contents of two of them and half of the third, then administered the drug. Within a few minutes, the patient's blood pressure dropped to 70/30 mm Hg and she became tachycardic.

Her doctor was summoned to the ICU. As soon as he saw the empty vials of hydralazine near the patient's bed, he realized she'd been given an overdose. A rapid infusion of I.V. fluids raised her blood pressure to a safe level.

Telephone orders can be misunderstood for many reasons. But taking certain precautions can resolve any misunderstandings *before* a drug is given.

First, always repeat the order back to the doctor, pronouncing each digit of the dose. For example, "That's 50 milligrams, five-zero milligrams, of Vistaril?" Or "You want 17 units, one-seven units, of regular insulin?"

Second, remember that a single dose of a drug will rarely amount to more than two dose units, whether they be vials, ampules, tablets, or capsules. If you've obtained more than two units for a single dose, double-check the order with the doctor. There's a good chance someone's made an error.

Notes:

Error
Number

104

Giving a drug in the wrong diluent

A young man hospitalized for uncontrolled diabetes developed cardiac dysrhythmias. His doctor ordered a lidocaine (lignocaine) drip: 2 grams in 500 ml of 0.9% sodium chloride for injection. The nurse quickly obtained a premixed solution containing the correct concentration of lidocaine and hung it for the patient. Unfortunately, she didn't read the label closely. If she had, she would have seen that the lidocaine was diluted not in sodium chloride but in 5% *dextrose* for injection. The patient was spared a possible hyperglycemic episode because another nurse stopped the infusion when she realized what it contained.

Premixed intravenous solutions are available for many commonly used drugs, including heparin, cimetidine, and numerous antibiotics. These solutions save nursing time and can help prevent medication errors because the proper dose of the correct drug has already been added. But using them doesn't eliminate the need to give all labels a careful reading.

Don't repeat this nurse's mistake. When obtaining a premixed solution, compare both the drug *and* diluent listed on the label with the doctor's order. When it comes to administering medications in this form, the right diluent is just as important as the right drug.

Notes: _____

_____

_____

_____

_____

Using outdated measurements

A woman with a history of peptic ulcer disease was admitted to a long-term care facility. Her doctor ordered Maalox, 30 ml, 1 hour before meals and at bedtime. The nurse who transcribed the order used the apothecary symbol for fluidounce (see below)—or so she thought. What she actually used was the symbol for fluidram (see below), which is equivalent to 5 ml. Consequently, the patient was given only 5-ml doses for several days. The error was discovered when another nurse questioned the low dose.

Granted, this is not an earthshaking medication error. But think what could have happened had the order been for oral theophylline, morphine, or cyclosporine. The patient could have been dangerously undermedicated. Or consider the consequences if the symbol for ounce had been written for dram: The patient would have received an overdose.

The apothecary system of measurement has long outlived its usefulness. It's confusing and hazardous. Many doctors and nurses interchange the abbreviations for ounce and dram in drug orders. They mistake the designation minim (see below) for ml. And they confuse grains and grams.

Yet some nursing schools still teach the apothecary system. Doctors persist in using it in their orders. Even drug companies promote its use. A minim scale still appears on some syringes, and doses in grains remain on some manufacturers' labels (for example, labels for sublingual nitroglycerin tablets).

Don't let the apothecary system put your patients at risk. Discourage its use whenever you can. For drug doses, metric is the only way to go.

fluidounce   **fluidram**   **minim**

Notes:

_____

_____

_____

_____

_____

Improperly mixing I.V. additives

A man who'd been vomiting for several days was admitted to the hospital emergency department (ED) for dehydration. There, the ED nurse started an infusion of D_5W.

When the patient's doctor arrived, he asked the nurse to add 40 mEq of potassium chloride (KCl) to the patient's I.V. bag. The nurse carried out the order. Instantly, the patient cried out in pain, saying he felt a burning sensation going up his arm. The nurse stopped the infusion immediately and the pain subsided.

The doctor suspected that the nurse hadn't added the KCl properly. He'd seen reports in the literature about KCl pooling when it was added to a hanging, flexible plastic I.V. bag. When that happened, the patient essentially got a bolus of KCl, an extremely dangerous—and irritating—substance. A bolus of this drug will cause intense pain at the infusion site and in the vein. It also creates the risk of transient hyperkalemia, which could lead to dysrhythmias.

When the doctor inquired, the nurse claimed she injected the KCl slowly, then had gently squeezed the bag. This confirmed the doctor's suspicions that the drug hadn't been thoroughly mixed into the solution.

Pooling of a drug additive can occur when: (1) the bag is hanging with the injection port straight down; (2) the drug is added slowly; and (3) the needle of the syringe containing the additive is only partially inserted into the bag's injection port. Unless the bag is inverted several times to mix the solution, the drug could concentrate near the fluid exit port.

To prevent improper mixing, avoid adding medications to I.V. solutions that are already infusing. Ask your hospital to develop policies whereby a new container must be prepared and hung. If you have no alternative, follow these guidelines:
• Close the roller clamp on the I.V. line or turn the infusion pump off.
• Insert the syringe needle *completely* into the bag, up to the needle hub. Be sure to use a 1½-inch needle. Using a shorter needle or inserting it only partially into the port can cause pooling of the additive.
• Inject the additive *quickly*. If the injection takes more than 5 seconds, it could cause pooling.
• After injecting the additive, remove the bag from the I.V. pole and invert it at least three times. Just squeezing or shaking the bag isn't enough to mix the drug into the solution.

Not knowing what form of a drug is being given and why

After receiving a liver transplant, a 31-year-old woman with impaired renal function developed pneumonia. Her doctor ordered I.V. vancomycin (Vancocin) to treat one of the causative organisms, a resistant staphylococcus. To protect the patient's renal function, he ordered the drug given every 96 hours.

Weeks later, while still receiving I.V. vancomycin, the patient developed pseudomembranous enterocolitis. The infectious disease specialist recommended oral vancomycin. The intern, thinking the oral drug would replace the I.V. drug, ordered the I.V. vancomycin discontinued and oral vancomycin given instead.

Unfortunately, the intern didn't know that each of these two forms of vancomycin has a specific indication. Oral vancomycin effectively treats pseudomembranous enterocolitis, but is *not* effective for systemic infections because it's not absorbed when taken by mouth. And I.V. vancomycin, which is effective against systemic infections, won't treat pseudomembranous enterocolitis. The patient needed both forms of the drug.

The error went unnoticed for some time because the I.V. vancomycin had been given so infrequently. When the patient's regular doctor discovered what had happened, he ordered an immediate I.V. bolus of vancomycin, followed by resumption of the original I.V. regimen. The patient pulled through and was eventually discharged.

A series of assumptions led to this error. One, the infectious disease specialist assumed that the intern knew to continue the I.V. drug. Two, the intern (and the patient's nurses) assumed that the oral drug could replace the I.V. drug. And three, the pharmacist who reviewed the intern's order assumed that the patient no longer needed the I.V. drug.

Don't let assumptions endanger your patients. Know what you're giving and why.

Notes:

_____

_____

_____

_____

_____

Error
Number

108

Giving an excess dose because of a confusing abbreviation

A doctor wrote an order for Lasix, 40 mg, 1 O.D. He meant for the diuretic to be given once daily. But a new nurse thought the period after the "O" was a slash mark and interpreted the order as "10/D." So she gave the patient *ten* 40-mg tablets daily.

Within a few days, the patient became dehydrated and developed an electrolyte imbalance. The error was discovered when the nurse overheard the doctor say he never expected such problems with only 40 mg of Lasix. The nurse told him the patient had been receiving 400 mg.

This error offers two lessons. First, if you have to give more than two tablets, capsules, ampules, or other form of a drug to complete a dose, check with the pharmacist or doctor. A mistake has probably been made. Second, don't accept abbreviations for "daily." The abbreviation "O.D." could also be read as "right eye"—a potentially dangerous misinterpretation if the drug is a liquid. The designation "q.d." could be interpreted as "q.i.d.," and "1/d." could be seen as "t.i.d."

Notes:

Failing to specify on the MAR if the doctor orders two tablets

A patient hospitalized for fainting spells was found to have frequent premature ventricular contractions. Her doctor ordered two tablets of quinidine gluconate (Quinaglute), an antiarrhythmic, given every 8 hours. Quinaglute is available only in 324-mg tablets. So the nurse who transcribed the order onto the patient's medication administration record (MAR) wrote it this way:

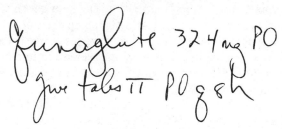

During the night shift, the medication nurse prepared to administer this patient's drugs. She glanced at the MAR and saw "Quinaglute, 324 mg." Thinking just one tablet was called for, she pulled apart the two unit-dose packages that had been taped together by the pharmacist and used only one of them. The pharmacist discovered the error in the morning when he found the leftover tablet in the patient's drug bin.

This error could have been prevented if the nurse transcribing the order had clearly stated two tablets were needed: *Quinaglute, 648 mg (2 x 324-mg tablets), q8h*. Also, the medication nurse should have stopped to consider why the two packages were taped together. Most pharmacists using a unit-dose system will do this (or leave the packages unperforated) when an order requires more than one dose unit.

Notes:

_____

_____

_____

_____

_____

Error
Number

110

Accidentally reversing infusion bags when replacing them on the pumps

A 78-year-old woman on an intensive care unit was receiving intravenous nitroglycerin and lidocaine (lignocaine) to treat angina and congestive heart failure. Her nurses carefully titrated the medications, using a separate infusion pump for each. To avoid confusion, the nurses labeled each pump with the name and concentration of the drug being infused.

One morning, just before change of shift, the night-shift nurse replaced the two infusion bags and their tubing according to hospital protocol. Shortly after the day-shift nurses arrived, the patient complained of angina. Her nurse increased the rate of the nitroglycerin infusion, but the patient still had pain. Soon she became lethargic and confused.

The nurse called the patient's doctor, who suspected lidocaine toxicity. Discontinuing the lidocaine, he too increased the rate of the nitroglycerin infusion.

By this time, the patient was stuporous, but still mumbling about chest pain. Suspecting she'd taken a turn for the worse, the nurse called in the family.

Just then, another nurse discovered what was wrong. The night-shift nurse had accidentally reversed the infusion bags when replacing them on the pumps. Nobody had read the labels on the bags; instead, they had assumed the labels on the pumps were correct. As a result, the patient had been receiving increasing amounts of lidocaine and no nitroglycerin. She was indeed experiencing a toxic reaction to the lidocaine.

The doctor ordered the lidocaine temporarily stopped and the nitroglycerin restarted. Within a few hours, the patient was responsive and free of pain.

You can imagine how serious such an error could be. Never rely on an infusion pump's label: Read the label on the infusion container. And when checking the patient's infusion or making any adjustments to the setup, trace it from the container, to the pump, to the patient.

Notes:

Confusing "I.U." with "I.V."

Vitamin D_2 liquid (Drisdol), 50,000 I.U. daily, was ordered for a woman who had hypoparathyroidism. Both the unit secretary who transcribed the order and the nurse who reviewed it mistook the abbreviation "I.U." (international units) for "I.V." (intravenous). And that's how the drug was scheduled.

Later, when the pharmacist sent up a dose of Drisdol in an oral syringe, the nurse thought he'd made an error. She discovered her mistake when she called to ask why the drug wasn't in an I.V. syringe.

This near miss could have been prevented if the doctor had made it clear in his order that the medication was to be administered orally. Also, he could have simply written "units"; the "I" for "international" really isn't needed. In any event, keep in mind that you'll see the abbreviation "I.U." used in certain orders. Don't confuse it with "I.V."

Notes:

_____

_____

_____

_____

Error
Number

112

Not verifying abnormal lab values

A laboratory technician called to report a low serum potassium level of 2.4 mEq/liter for Mrs. Johnson, a newly admitted diabetic patient. (Normal range is 3.8 to 5.5 mEq/liter.) The unit secretary who took the call notified the charge nurse and, when the computer printout of the result was run, placed it on Mrs. Johnson's chart.

The nurse checked the lab value against the printout and called the patient's doctor. Although he was surprised by the report, he ordered an I.V. infusion of potassium chloride, 60 mEq/liter, to be given over 8 hours during the night. He also ordered another serum potassium test done in the morning.

The next morning, Mrs. Johnson's potassium level was 6.6 mEq/liter. As the nurse was calling the doctor to report this abnormally high level, she glanced at the previous day's printout and saw that the patient name wasn't Johnson but *Jackson*. The unit secretary had apparently heard the name wrong on the phone and hadn't checked it on the printout.

Mrs. Johnson needed several 30-gram doses of oral Kayexalate over the next 2 days to bring her serum potassium level back to normal. And Mrs. Jackson required immediate potassium supplementation.

Such potentially dangerous errors needn't happen. Verify abnormal lab values before taking steps to treat them. Just as important: Read the patient's name on every computer printout and compare it with the name on the chart.

Notes:

Confusing a vial of Demerol with a saline solution flush

A busy nurse was preparing to give an I.V. antibiotic to one of her patients. She obtained the premixed minibag and attached it to the patient's I.V. set.

At the same time, another nurse withdrew a Tubex of meperidine (Demerol), 100 mg, from the drug cart's narcotic drawer. Seeing that a dose of hydroxyzine (Vistaril) was supposed to be given at the same time, she set the Demerol on top of the cart while she went to get the other drug.

Meanwhile, the first nurse remembered that she needed to flush her patient's I.V. line before giving the antibiotic. She came out to the drug cart and, seeing the Tubex lying on top of it, picked it up, thinking it was a saline flush. She then proceeded to inject the 100 mg of Demerol into the patient's heparin lock.

The patient immediately developed respiratory distress and had no audible blood pressure or palpable pulse. The nurse read the label and realized what she'd done. She called a code. The patient was given naloxone (Narcan) and was revived.

Two commonsense rules can help prevent such errors:
• *Never* leave any medication unattended.
• *Always* read the label on a medication before you give it; don't rely on its appearance. Make this rule second nature when administering drugs.

Notes:

_____

_____

_____

_____

_____

Not knowing how to use the endotracheal route in an emergency

A 47-year-old man who'd suffered a cardiac arrest was taken to an emergency department. A code was called. Team members intubated the patient successfully, but they couldn't find a vein for fluid and drug administration.

The code doctor decided to perform a venous cutdown, but he didn't want to delay administering epinephrine. So he elected to give this drug by the endotracheal route.

The doctor handed a syringe of epinephrine, with the needle removed, to a nurse, telling her to "put this in the endotracheal tube." The nurse had never given a drug by this route before. She hesitated a moment, then attached the syringe to the access site for inflating the cuff.

Fortunately, the nurse anesthetist saw what the nurse was doing and stopped her. The anesthetist then correctly instilled the epinephrine directly into the endotracheal tube.

Endotracheal administration of drugs in an emergency has become fairly common, but not everyone is familiar with the procedure. To instill a drug correctly by this route, use sodium chloride injection or sterile water for injection to dilute the drug to a volume of 10 to 25 ml. (This volume appears to provide the best absorption in the shortest amount of time.) Instill the solution into the tube, then follow instillation with several insufflations of air.

Drugs that can be given this way include epinephrine, lidocaine (lignocaine), atropine, and naloxone. Others may be added to the list as endotracheal administration becomes even more common.

Don't be caught unprepared in an emergency. Know how to use the endotracheal route, and make sure your colleagues know the procedure as well.

Notes:

_____

_____

_____

_____

_____

Forgetting to release the clamp on the tubing for I.V. drug administration

During medication rounds one evening, a nurse hung an I.V. minibag containing the antibiotic cefoxitin (Mefoxin) for a diabetic teenager who had cellulitis of the right foot. The infusion was scheduled to start at 6 p.m. and finish infusing within a half hour.

When the night-shift nurse went to hang a second minibag at midnight, she found that the first bag was still full. The reason was simple—the evening nurse had forgotten to release the clamp from the tubing.

Needless to say, I.V. drug administration isn't complete until you check the solution to make sure it's infusing properly. This rule holds true whether you're using a gravity set or an electronic infusion control device. Had the evening nurse checked the infusion after she'd hung it, she could have discovered her oversight and corrected it.

Remember the basics: Check all new infusions within 10 minutes after starting them. And when checking, assess the entire system—from the bag to the I.V. site.

Notes:

<table>
<tr>
<td>

Error
Number

116

</td>
<td>

Not clarifying the abbreviation "p.c."

A 64-year-old woman was hospitalized for treatment of rheumatoid arthritis. Her doctor wrote the following order for the antiinflammatory drug Feldene (piroxicam):

Feldene 20 mg PO pc

Both the patient's nurse and the hospital pharmacist interpreted the "p.c." to mean "after each meal," and that's how the drug was scheduled.

The patient was given Feldene three times a day for more than a week. Then she began vomiting blood. Studies revealed severe anemia and a peptic ulcer. The doctor ordered several units of blood administered, then set out to find the cause of the bleeding.

His search didn't take long. As soon as he reviewed the patient's medication administration record, he saw that she was being given Feldene three times a day, not once a day as he had intended. He was well aware that this drug can cause bleeding, even when given no more than once daily as recommended. The doctor discontinued the Feldene and prescribed drug therapy for the patient's ulcer.

The doctor, nurse, and pharmacist all contributed to this error. The abbreviation "p.c." commonly means "after a meal." The doctor wrote an incomplete order by not specifying after *which* meal or noting that the drug was to be given only once a day. The nurse and pharmacist transcribed, filled, and carried out the order mechanically, without considering that it was incomplete. Ironically, both said later that they knew Feldene shouldn't be given more than once daily. But when they reviewed the order, they were so busy they didn't give it a second thought.

Don't let a hectic pace cause an error. When you're especially busy, review drug orders even more diligently. Think each order through, and clarify those that are incomplete.

</td>
</tr>
</table>

Being unfamiliar with crash cart drugs

A code was called for a patient who'd developed ventricular fibrillation. After the patient had been stabilized, the doctor decided to replace the lidocaine (lignocaine) infusion that was running with one containing procainamide. He asked the nurse to add 1 gram of the drug to 500 ml of D_5W injection.

The nurse searched the crash cart and found a 10-ml vial of procainamide. When she read the label, she thought it indicated that the vial contained 100 mg of procainamide. She drew up the contents into a syringe and began looking for additional vials.

Just then, the doctor called for a 100-mg bolus of procainamide. The nurse handed him the syringe. As the doctor started to inject the drug, the nurse read the vial label again and realized what it *really* said: 100 mg per *milliliter,* not per vial. She stopped the doctor from completing the injection.

Such an error points up the importance of familiarizing yourself with the contents of the crash cart *before* a code is called. If you see a drug label that's confusing, alert the pharmacist. He may be able to replace it with one that's less confusing. He may also be able to supply only single-dose containers. If a multidose vial must be used, he can add a cautionary label.

Notes:

Error
Number

118

Inadvertently administering medications or liquid feedings in the wrong catheter, tube, or body cavity

A 78-year-old stroke victim who couldn't swallow had a gastrostomy tube inserted for liquid feedings. She also had an indwelling urinary catheter.

To control diarrhea caused by the tube feedings, her doctor ordered a kaolin-pectin mixture (Kaopectate). During shift change, a nurse was puzzled by the milky white fluid in the patient's urinary collection bag.

Here's what happened. Earlier in the day, a medication nurse had turned off the feeding pump and disconnected what she thought was the gastrostomy tube. She instilled the Kaopectate, then reconnected the catheter to restart the feeding. What she'd actually done was put the Kaopectate into the patient's urinary catheter, not the gastrostomy tube. The medication went directly into the patient's bladder.

The nurse who discovered the mistake called the patient's doctor, who ordered a bladder irrigation and antibiotics. The patient's urinary catheter and collection bag were replaced.

Occasionally we hear about nurses who inadvertently administer medications or liquid feedings in the wrong catheter, tube, or body cavity. These errors may cause serious injuries—even death. So play it safe: Always trace a length of tubing from its distal to its proximal end. Better yet, label all tubing so that it's virtually impossible to get two lengths of tubing mixed up. And make sure unnecessary tubes are discontinued as early as possible.

Notes:

_____

_____

_____

_____

_____

Neglecting to question an unusually high dose of penicillin

A nurse noticed that a postpartum patient with a relatively minor infection was scheduled to receive an unusually high dose of penicillin:

Penicillin 6.5 million units

Thinking that another nurse had transcribed the order incorrectly, she looked at the original on the patient's chart and discovered a dangerous misinterpretation. The doctor's sloppy handwriting made the "G" after penicillin look like a 6. And he had written the 500,000 units as ".5 million units," instead of "0.5 million units." So the order *did* look like 6.5 million units.

The nurse called the doctor, who confirmed that he really wanted his patient to have only 500,000 units every 4 hours—a total of 3,000,000 units a day.

The doctor and the nurse who transcribed the order share the blame for this error. The doctor should have been more careful when he wrote the order. If he had put a zero in front of the decimal point and used the drug's proper name, penicillin G potassium, the order would have been clear.

The first nurse, though, should have realized that the apparent dose was much too high. Although it occasionally causes a serious allergic reaction, penicillin G is a very safe drug. But because each million units contains 1.7 mEq of potassium, a mistake in the administration rate or the dose could be fatal for a child or for an adult with a serious illness.

Notes:

_____

_____

_____

_____

Error
Number

120

Not guarding against human error

A nurse took a pharmacy-prepared I.V. piggyback dose of cefazolin (Ancef), 1 gram, from the refrigerator. She checked the computer label, which included the patient's name, room number, and medication order. Then, she rechecked it against the patient's medication administration record. Before administering the antibiotic, she also verified the patient's identity. Everything appeared to be in order.

The next day the nurse's manager told her that an incident report had been filled out because the patient had received the wrong drug. The mistake had been discovered by the nurse on the next shift. She was about to give the patient another dose of the antibiotic when she realized that the pharmacist had erroneously placed the patient's label on a bag of ampicillin. The original label—the one the pharmacist had put on the bag when he had originally mixed the I.V. that morning—was visible.

You rely on the pharmacy to dispense drugs accurately, and a degree of trust is essential. But don't trust blindly. Check all labels on any container or I.V. bag.

Human error is always possible. Trust...but also verify.

Notes:

Relying on medication box labels instead of on container labels

An 8-year-old diabetic patient who had developed ketoacidosis was admitted to an emergency department. As one nurse drew blood for glucose levels and other laboratory tests, another nurse took an I.V. bag from a box labeled "sodium chloride injection" and started an I.V. infusion. She also administered insulin.

When the first nurse finished drawing blood, she looked up at the I.V. container and noticed that it was dextrose injection—the last thing a diabetic patient in ketoacidosis needs. The nurse immediately clamped the line, found the correct solution, and hung it. Luckily, only a small amount of dextrose had been infused.

Don't rely on the labels on boxes to identify drugs or I.V. solutions. Someone may have put the drug or solution in the wrong box. (The same goes for labeled trays, drawers, or shelves.) The only reliable way to identify a drug or solution is by reading the immediate *container* label.

Notes:

Error
Number

122

Not taking the time to assure that infusions are set up properly

A patient on an intensive care unit was receiving both lidocaine (lignocaine, Xylocaine) and nitroglycerin infusions. When his nurse turned him on his side to auscultate his posterior breath sounds, she discovered that the needle attached to the nitroglycerin piggyback line had been dislodged from the male adapter cap and was soaking the bed. The patient wasn't injured, but he wasn't receiving his nitroglycerin either. The nurse changed the needle and restarted the infusion.

When a patient is receiving piggybacked I.V. medications, take a few extra seconds to tape the needle in the Y-site cap or male adapter cap. This will help prevent the needle from coming loose and ensure that the patient receives his medication.

Notes:

Using decimal points on medication orders when they serve no purpose

A doctor ordered oral warfarin for a patient with a history of phlebitis. In the past, this patient needed only small doses of warfarin to stabilize her condition. So the doctor prescribed an initial dose of 1 mg. But when he wrote the order, he put a decimal point after the 1 and added a 0. Unfortunately, a line on the order form obscured the decimal point. To the pharmacist who received a copy of the order, and to the unit secretary and nurse who kept the original, the order looked like *10* mg. That's what the patient received.

Two days later, the patient's prothrombin time was 38 seconds. (Her control time was 12 seconds.) The doctor ordered phytonadione (vitamin K_1, AquaMEPHYTON) to reverse the effects of the overdose.

This error could have been avoided if the doctor had simply written the order as 1 mg, not 1.0 mg. The decimal point and the zero serve no purpose. The order can easily be misinterpreted, especially if the decimal point is hard to see or, as in this case, if it's on top of a line on the order form. (These lines on a form, by the way, may also cut off the tops of 7s, so they end up looking like 1s.)

A carbonless form with lines only on the original may also have prevented this error. If there were no lines on his copy, the pharmacist probably would have noticed the decimal point and dispensed the correct dose. But the easiest solution is to simply eliminate unnecessary decimal points and zeros.

Notes:

Error Number	**Administering concentrated sodium chloride solution instead of normal saline solution**

124

A nursing instructor agreed to be the "guinea pig" for a student who needed practice giving intradermal skin tests. The instructor suggested that they use 0.1 ml of sodium chloride injection. They found a fresh vial on the nursing unit, and the student flawlessly prepared and administered the intradermal injection. The instructor, though, felt an unusual burning at the injection site. She and the student rechecked the vial, but everything seemed to be in order.

Two days later, the instructor noticed sloughing and ulceration around the site. She found another vial with the same label and took it to the hospital pharmacist. He examined it and identified the solution as *concentrated* sodium chloride injection, 146 mg/ml (14.6%, 2.5 mEq/ml). She should have used 0.9% sodium chloride injection (normal saline).

Concentrated sodium chloride injection shouldn't be kept on a nursing unit. (The exception is a hemodialysis unit, where it's used to elevate blood volume and reverse hyponatremia.) Vials of the concentrated solution are used to prepare I.V. admixtures in the pharmacy.

The instructor and her student learned an important lesson about reading labels carefully and completely before giving any medication. If they had, they would have seen the warning label that's found on all vials of concentrated sodium chloride: *"Must be diluted prior to I.V. administration."*

Pharmacists should be careful to place stocks of concentrated sodium chloride injection in special storage areas. And they should consider adding warning labels over the caps of each vial.

Notes:

_____

_____

_____

_____

_____

Confusing drugs that are spelled or pronounced similarly

A patient with hypertension called her doctor's office to report dizziness and a headache. She told the nurse who took the call that these symptoms had started after her last visit to the doctor.

According to the patient's chart, the doctor had called in an order for Nimodipine (used to treat stroke) to the pharmacy. The nurse asked the patient to read the label on her bottle of pills. Instead of Nimodipine, the patient spelled out Nicardopine (used to treat hypertension). Nimodipine and Nicardopine sound pretty much the same. Apparently, the pharmacist thought the doctor had said Nimodipine when he'd called in the order.

Many pairs of drugs are spelled or pronounced alike. To prevent mix-ups, doctors should make it clear on the prescription *why* the patient needs to take the drug. If a doctor doesn't do that, the nurse and pharmacist should make sure they know why the drug is being prescribed before administering or dispensing it. Then, in most cases, they can be sure the drug is appropriate for the patient's condition.

Of course, asking doctors to spell the names of drugs may help, too, especially if you know two drugs are spelled or pronounced similarly.

Notes:
_____

_____

_____

_____

_____

Error
Number

126

Using outdated drug abbreviations

A doctor asked his resident to order AZT (azidothymidine),
200 mg, every 4 hours, for one of his patients. Azidothymidine
is the old name for zidovudine (Retrovir), the drug used to treat
signs and symptoms of acquired immunodeficiency syndrome
(AIDS). The resident mistakenly ordered azathioprine (Imuran),
an immunosuppressant normally given to transplant patients before and after surgery. The unit secretary entered the order into
the medication administration record, then forwarded it to the
pharmacy.

The pharmacist questioned the order when he realized that an
AIDS patient shouldn't be receiving an immunosuppressant. The
dosage was wrong, too—azathioprine is usually given once a
day, not every 4 hours. The pharmacist called the nursing unit;
the patient's nurse located the doctor, who clarified the order.
The patient received the correct drug.

Using the current names for the AIDS drug—zidovudine or
Retrovir—instead of the old abbreviation AZT would prevent this
kind of mix-up. In fact, hospitals should ban abbreviations for all
drugs, except for those that are well-established and appear on an
approved hospital list (like MOM for milk of magnesia).

Notes: _____

_____

_____

_____

_____

Confusing "magnesium sulfate" with "morphine sulfate"

A new graduate nurse was working in an emergency department (ED) when she received an order for "M.S. 5 mg." She stood in front of the medication cabinet for several minutes searching for a drug with the initials "M.S." She found magnesium sulfate, which she took to the doctor. When she showed him the vial, he told her she had the wrong medication; he wanted morphine sulfate.

Obviously, the nurse should have asked him what he wanted before she went to the medication cabinet. If you don't understand an abbreviation, admit it—don't be too intimidated or embarrassed to ask.

This problem brings up another point: Don't use an abbreviation unless it's on the hospital's approved list. Most of us would know that an ED doctor wanted morphine sulfate when he asked for "M.S.," but a new graduate or a float nurse might not. And that could result in a serious error.

Notes:

_____

_____

_____

_____

_____

Error
Number

128

Relying on a vial's appearance rather than its label

A hemodialysis nurse discovered that the unit had exhausted its stock of 50-ml vials of mannitol 25% injection. (According to the unit's protocol, nurses administered mannitol to increase blood volume when a dialysis patient became hypotensive.) The nurse checked the backup supply and took a vial from the shelf where the mannitol was usually stored. Then she drew up the contents of the vial and injected the drug into a hypotensive patient. Almost instantly, he went into cardiac arrest. The nurse started cardiopulmonary resuscitation, but the patient died.

After the patient's death, nurses on the unit realized that he'd received mannitol from the backup supply, so they checked the discarded vial. It had contained lidocaine (lignocaine, Xylocaine), not mannitol. Both drugs were in 50-ml vials sealed with light-blue caps. After she removed the vial from the shelf, the nurse failed to read the label. She'd simply chosen the vial for its size, shape, and position on the shelf.

We all know the hazards of failing to read labels, but sooner or later someone will make this type of mistake. And, as in this case, a tragedy sometimes occurs.

But we can minimize the risk of error if we're on the lookout for potential hazards—and if we suggest ways to correct them. For example, a hemodialysis unit stocks Xylocaine to use as an anesthetic. But why in 50-ml vials? Smaller ampules or vials—say, 5 ml or 10 ml—would work just as well. If such a policy had been in effect, the nurse wouldn't have relied on the vial's appearance. Even if she had, the dose in a smaller vial would have been less likely to cause cardiac arrest.

Notes:

_____

_____

_____

_____

_____

Keeping vials of potassium chloride on a bedside table

A cancer patient who was about to be discharged asked a nurse to watch her husband irrigate her Hickman catheter. As the nurse watched, the husband carefully drew up the correct amount of solution and performed the irrigation properly.

Within seconds, the patient went into cardiac arrest. Despite resuscitative measures, she died.

The nurses discovered that the husband had picked up a vial of potassium chloride instead of heparin. But they couldn't figure out why potassium chloride was on the bedside table. Normally, it was kept in the unit's stock to prepare I.V. admixtures when the pharmacy was closed.

This tragedy needn't have occurred. If the nurse had noticed that the husband hadn't read the container label—or if she'd read it first—she could have prevented the error.

But as with most medication errors, she wasn't the only one to blame. Nurse-managers should keep that in mind when they're reviewing errors at the hospitals where they work. When we search for a lone scapegoat, we may miss other things that contributed to the error. And that means the mistake may occur again.

Let's look at the other factors that contributed to this error. A vial of potassium chloride shouldn't be left on a bedside table, of course. But did it even need to be on the unit? If the hospital couldn't keep the pharmacy's I.V. admixture service open around the clock, perhaps the pharmacist could have provided premixed, commercially available containers of potassium chloride in common I.V. solutions. Or the potassium chloride could have been in a controlled storage area, a step some hospitals are taking.

This hospital used heparin and potassium chloride from the same manufacturer. The vials stocked on the unit were similar in size, shape, and color, as were their labels. The pharmacy could have substituted another brand for either one or used a smaller vial. Heparin, for example, is available in 1-ml and 5-ml vials and in prefilled syringes.

We can easily think of ways to avert a tragedy after it has happened. Blaming one person or one thing won't fix what's wrong. We have to look at the whole picture and consider changes that could prevent a fatal error.

Error
Number

130

Accepting a substitute for a written order

A medical/surgical nurse who had floated to the emergency department admitted an 18-month-old boy suffering from an acute asthma attack. A doctor called out an order for atropine, 0.25 mg, to be given intramuscularly. The nurse repeated the order to the doctor, then rushed to prepare the dose. When she passed the doctor in the hallway, she repeated the order. He again confirmed it.

After she administered the drug, the nurse charted the order and showed it to the doctor. He told her she'd just given the child an overdose. What he'd meant to say was 0.025 mg (not 0.25) of atropine. Fortunately, the child experienced only intense flushing.

The doctor apologized for yelling out the incorrect order, but that was little consolation for the nurse, who realized she'd made a potentially serious error.

She and her colleagues learned a valuable lesson that's become a hospital policy: A doctor can't give—and a nurse can't accept—a verbal order when the doctor is on the unit. He has to write it on the patient's chart. The only exceptions are code emergencies or when the doctor is actively performing a procedure.

And the nurse learned that she should always look up and confirm doses—or at least double-check them with another knowledgeable professional—when she's unfamiliar with a drug.

Notes:

Misreading "OJ" as "OU"

A doctor ordered the expectorant saturated solution of potassium iodide (SSKI), 10 drops in "OJ" (orange juice), to be given four times a day to a patient with pneumonia. The new graduate nurse read the handwritten order and proceeded to instill 10 drops of SSKI in each of the patient's eyes.

How could a drug that should be diluted in orange juice and given orally end up in someone's eyes? It's not so outlandish when you consider what happened: The nurse misread the sloppily written abbreviation "OJ" as "OU" (each eye). She must have assumed SSKI was an irrigating fluid for the eyes. Unfortunately, the patient developed chemical conjunctivitis.

This kind of mistake happens more often than you might think. Consider these examples of how OJ could be misread:

$$OJ \qquad OD \qquad OS$$

Besides the obvious remedy—avoiding the abbreviation OJ—you can ask your pharmacist to do one of two things: Label dropper bottles of SSKI with "For oral use only" or "Do not use in eyes," or supply a prediluted potassium iodide solution that negates the need for orange juice.

Notes:

_____

_____

_____

_____

Error Number	**Not taking additional precautions with home I.V. therapy**
132	

A home care nurse visited a patient to change his pump cassette and reset his ambulatory infusion pump for a newly prescribed concentration of fluorouracil, an anticancer drug. She reprogrammed the pump incorrectly. Within 24 hours, the patient received a 5-day supply of the drug. He began vomiting repeatedly and eventually developed leukopenia. Luckily, he recovered.

Home I.V. therapy requires extra precautions. A patient at home won't receive the same close monitoring he would in the hospital. So you have to be especially vigilant when manipulating infusion control devices. Plus, the drugs commonly infused with ambulatory pumps—such as anticancer drugs, I.V. narcotics, and other critical care drugs—warrant special attention.

At least two people should check pump settings or changes to make sure the device has been programmed correctly. For example, when you know you're going to change a setting, you could ask the pharmacist for a pump that's set properly before you leave for the patient's home. Once there, you would change the pumps, returning the old one to the pharmacist.

Or, if the doctor orders a change while you're at the patient's home, you can calculate the dosage and setting change, then call the pharmacist or another home care nurse. During your call, you would review and verify the steps you've taken to reprogram the pump. As an extra precaution, you could read the pump settings from the LED screens.

You should also teach the patient what the settings should be. If he notices that they're off, he can alert you before a problem develops. But make sure the lockout feature is activated so the patient can't inadvertently change the settings.

These steps could drastically reduce the risk of harming a patient with an erroneous ambulatory pump setting.

Notes:

Reversing the dose of regular and NPH insulin

A nurse who was supposed to give a combined dose of NPH and regular insulin went to the refrigerator where insulin vials were stored. She took one vial from the NPH box and another from the regular box, then drew up 40 units of NPH and 6 units of regular. The solution should have been cloudy. But it was almost clear, so she suspected that something was wrong.

She examined the insulin vials and discovered that someone had placed them in the wrong boxes. So the nurse had actually drawn up 40 units of regular and 6 units of NPH insulin.

We've discussed this before, but it bears repeating: Don't rely on a vial's storage container or box, a shelf label, or the label on a bin or drawer. *Always read the label on the drug vial itself.* If possible, throw away the boxes and store only the vials.

Notes:

_____

_____

_____

_____

_____

Error
Number

134

Relying on only one health care professional to interpret a drug order

A pharmacist received this medication order:

Following standard procedure, the nurse who'd processed the doctor's order had also sent the pharmacist a copy of her transcription. In the section of the medication administration record (MAR) marked "orders," she'd incorrectly noted the frequency for the antibiotic Rocephin (which she—and the doctor—had spelled Rhocephin) as "q.i.d." The pharmacist called her immediately and told her to change the MAR entry to "q12h" before an error was made. Rocephin is normally given only once or twice a day.

This transcription error is a good example of how illegible handwriting causes problems and why at least two professionals—a nurse and a pharmacist—must interpret every drug order. Here, the nurse had misread the doctor's sloppily written "q12h" as "q.i.d." Plus, he'd spelled the drug's name incorrectly and she'd copied it that way. And because she hadn't suspected an error, she didn't consult the unit's drug handbook.

At some hospitals, only one person interprets orders. For example, the nurse may forward a transcription of the order—but not the original order—to the pharmacy. This most often occurs in critical care areas of the hospital, such as the operating room, emergency department, and intensive care unit. So the pharmacist won't necessarily know if she's made an error. Similarly, a problem might come up if a nurse doesn't double-check the pharmacist's work when he interprets the order and prepares a computerized MAR.

Luckily, the pharmacist caught this transcription error before the patient received twice the prescribed amount of Rocephin. That underscores the value of the nurse and pharmacist double-checking the original order.

Confusing "Suprol" with "Cipro"

A doctor called the nursing unit to order Suprol, 500 mg, one tablet b.i.d. When the nurse discovered that the drug wasn't available, she called him back. What he'd actually said was Cipro, 500 mg.

When taking a verbal order, repeat what you heard. Because many drug names sound alike, you should also spell the name of the drug to verify it.

Doctors should include a strength with the drug name to help you identify the drug—even if it's available in only one strength. Also, if you know the patient's diagnosis, you can prevent errors by making sure that the therapy makes sense for the patient. In this case, the doctor might have said, "one tablet b.i.d. for urinary tract infection."

Notes:

_____

_____

_____

_____

_____

Error
Number

136

Mistaking a vial of spinal fluid with a vial of glutaraldehyde

A patient was scheduled for surgery to remove a cancerous eye. Before the procedure, the anesthesiologist removed some spinal fluid to decrease intracranial pressure. He placed the fluid in a small vial, which he marked "S.F." (for "spinal fluid") and set aside to reinject after the surgery.

An ophthalmology resident who was supposed to do a biopsy entered the operating room (OR) to pick up the eye. The surgeon hadn't yet removed it, so the resident said he'd come back later. Before leaving, he placed an unlabeled vial of glutaraldehyde—a formaldehyde-like preservative—on a table in the OR.

A nurse noticed the vial the resident had left behind and asked what was in it. Thinking she was referring to the vial the anesthesiologist had used, the surgeon told her it was spinal fluid. Because she didn't want an unlabeled vial in the OR, the nurse marked it accordingly.

After the operation was successfully completed, the patient was turned on his side to have the spinal fluid reinjected. Forgetting that he'd filled only one vial, the anesthesiologist injected the contents of both vials. The patient immediately went into cardiopulmonary arrest. During the resuscitation, the resident returned and asked where his vial of glutaraldehyde was. The cause of the arrest was then apparent. The patient died later that day.

Unlabeled vials or syringes containing any substance should never be left in a patient care area—or anywhere else. To do so is to invite a tragic error like this one. Nurse-managers should discuss this matter with the pharmacy and laboratory to make sure appropriate labels are provided.

Notes:

_____

_____

_____

_____

_____

Confusing "hydroxyzine" with "hydralazine"

A patient was scheduled to receive an intramuscular (I.M.) injection of 75 mg of meperidine (Demerol) mixed with 50 mg of hydroxyzine (Vistaril) every 4 hours as needed for pain. Because this patient was also severely hypertensive, the doctor had written a p.r.n. order for hydralazine (Apresoline), 20 mg I.M.

As in most hospitals, the pharmacist frequently dispensed generic drugs. So generic forms of Vistaril and Apresoline were in the patient's drug bin.

One afternoon, a nurse was preparing the injection of Demerol and Vistaril. She noticed that the vial of medication she thought was the generic equivalent of Vistaril contained a 20-mg dose. She needed 50 mg, which is how the Vistaril had previously been dispensed. A co-worker was also puzzled at first. Then she noticed that the vial contained *hydralazine,* not hydroxyzine.

When the pharmacy substitutes a generic drug for a drug that was ordered by its trade name, you must double-check to make sure you've got the right drug. If you're unfamiliar with generic equivalents, you should have a drug reference book handy.

Your pharmacist could help, too. When permitted by law, he could include both the generic and the trade names on labels and computer-generated medication administration records. In some states, this is considered misbranding, though. Others allow the pharmacist to make statements like "similar to Vistaril" or "substitute for Vistaril."

Also, the pharmacist can notify you of appropriate inventory changes. And unit-dose packaging will ensure that the dispensed medication retains its identity until you're ready to use it.

Notes:

_____

_____

_____

_____

Error
Number

138

Injecting medication into the wrong tube

A patient had an epidural catheter for intermittent morphine injections and a central line for I.V. fluids and other drugs. Neither catheter was labeled. Confusing the two lines, his nurse mistakenly injected 100 mg of furosemide (Lasix) into the epidural catheter. Fortunately, the patient wasn't harmed.

This error illustrates an all-too-common problem—the inadvertent injection of medication into the wrong tube. To prevent mix-ups like this, label all catheters at their distal ends. Also, trace each catheter from its insertion site to its most distal point, including the I.V. bag or bottle, before injecting a drug.

You can avoid potential errors by making sure that catheters—including nasogastric tubes, indwelling urinary catheters, and central lines—are in place only if absolutely necessary, or are disconnected as soon as possible.

Notes:

Storing nitroglycerin ointment incorrectly

After applying nitroglycerin ointment, a nurse accidentally left a tube of the ointment on her patient's bedside table. Later, she walked past the room and noticed the patient's wife rubbing something on his arm. When she investigated, she discovered that the wife was using the nitroglycerin ointment as a lotion. She quickly intervened and washed it off. Neither was harmed.

We occasionally hear of patients or family members who confuse nitroglycerin ointment with toothpaste or other ointments. When you send a patient home with nitroglycerin ointment, make sure you instruct him to store it away from look-alike tubes.

That's a good rule for you, too. Although you can't prevent a momentary lapse in thinking, as happened here, you can avoid storing nitroglycerin ointment incorrectly. For instance, don't leave it on top of the drug cart; a patient or family member could take it—deliberately or inadvertently—and misuse the drug.

Notes:

Error
Number

140

Confusing "Entex LA" with "Ex-Lax"

A patient with an eating disorder had just been admitted to the psychiatric unit. Before the nurse could assess her, an internist gave her a physical examination. He wrote this order:

$$\mathcal{E} \, a \, t \, \mathcal{E} \, x \, \mathcal{L} \, a \longrightarrow \div \, p o \, h i d$$

Both the nurse and the pharmacist interpreted the order as "eat Ex-Lax, one P.O. b.i.d." That didn't make sense, especially for a patient with an eating disorder. Before giving the Ex-Lax, the nurse consulted the attending psychiatrist. He was also puzzled by the order, so he discontinued it.

Neither the nurse nor the psychiatrist knew that during her physical the patient had complained of cold symptoms. The internist had actually ordered "Entex LA, one P.O. b.i.d." His sloppy handwriting had been misinterpreted. Unfortunately, the patient missed several doses of the decongestant-expectorant.

A more serious error—giving a laxative to a patient with an eating disorder—was avoided because the nurse knew her patient's diagnosis and the action of Ex-Lax. The internist could have helped by including more information with the original order. Many doctors aren't aware that indicating a drug's dosage form and its purpose can help nurses and pharmacists differentiate between drug names that look alike when handwritten. For example, a more complete order for Entex LA should have included "one tablet b.i.d. p.r.n. for cold symptoms." No one should have confused that for Ex-Lax.

Notes:

_____

_____

_____

_____

_____

Injecting an excessive dose because of failure to read the label

In a hospital emergency department (ED), a nurse needed to give 10,000 units of I.V. heparin to a patient who had just been diagnosed as having a pulmonary embolism. Normally, 5 ml vials of 1,000 units per ml were available in the ED. But this time, the nurse found a 5 ml vial that clearly listed "10,000" on the label right below the drug name. She drew up the entire contents and injected it I.V. into her patient.

Moments later, while hanging a follow-up heparin infusion container, another nurse came by with the empty vial and asked if the entire contents were injected. It turned out that the vial actually contained 10,000 units per ml. The volume she injected meant that she actually gave 50,000 units!

Looking at the vial more carefully, the nurse could see in small letters the words "units/ml" just below the 10,000. The vial's total volume was listed elsewhere on the label.

Although the nurse was at least partially to blame for not reading the label more carefully, the fact is that not all drug labels are as clear as they should be. Unless a manufacturer is extremely careful, he can unwittingly mislead users through malpositioning of important label information or by misuse of enhancements like boldface type, shaded backgrounds, colors, and size of type used for text.

In this case, the patient's physician felt that immediate administration of protamine sulfate, a heparin antagonist, was warranted. The patient suffered no sequelae.

To prevent such potentially fatal drug injections, be aware that labels can be misleading. Therefore, don't hurry such an important function as carefully reading the label. But you also need to do more. If you find yourself in a position of having to prepare an injection, make it a policy that at least another nurse or a physician double-check your work. Consider having both sets of initials on the medication administration record.

Finally, as a professional, you also have a responsibility to make some people aware of what you believe to be a misleading label. Let your pharmacist know so he can consider purchasing a less error prone product. And be sure to call the USP (they set labeling standards the FDA must follow) so they can in turn inform the manufacturer (1-800-638-6725).

Error
Number

142

Not making sure patients who are NPO have adequate fluid intake

A patient who was NPO following abdominal surgery was receiving dextrose 5% in water with ⅓ normal saline solution and 10 mEq of potassium chloride in each liter of I.V. fluid to run at 100 ml per hour. The doctor wrote an order reading:

*add 1 amp Berocca-C
to a liter of IV each day*

However, the nurse transcribing this vitamin order thought that the doctor intended for the infusion to be reduced to a liter of fluid over 24 hours. She wrote in the Kardex: *1 amp Berocca-C to 1,000 ml/day*. The label on the I.V. stand bottle in use still read: *run at 100 ml per hour*. But the nurse starting the new infusion reduced the rate to 50 ml per hour as indicated in the Kardex.

This error could have been avoided if the nurse who transcribed the order or the nurse who changed the flow rate had stopped to consider that the new rate meant that the patient, who was NPO, and had no other source of fluids, would have his fluid intake cut in half—a drastic change. Realizing this should have alerted them to double-check the medication order.

Notes:

Trying to fill in an order that doesn't include tablet strength

When a drug is available in only one strength, why bother to insist that the doctor specify strength in his medication order? Because drugs are sometimes marketed in strengths that you may be unaware of.

In one case, a doctor wrote this order:

[handwritten: Antivert tablet PO qid for dizziness]

A nurse noted the order in her records. Then, because she thought the drug came in only one strength, the nurse added *12.5-mg tablets* to the doctor's order and sent it to the pharmacy. The pharmacist saw the addition and assumed the nurse had checked tablet strength with the doctor.

Two days later, the doctor made rounds and saw that his patient wasn't responding well to the Antivert. When the nurse told him what dosage she'd been administering, the doctor told her he'd meant the patient to receive Antivert in a 25-mg tablet strength.

Clearly, the doctor could have avoided this error if he'd included tablet strength in his medication order. But when he didn't, the nurse should have checked with the doctor before she sent his order to the pharmacy.

Notes:

_____

_____

_____

_____

_____

Error
Number

144

Not making sure new nurses know how to administer medications

In most hospitals, new nurses must take written tests to establish their overall competence. But, sometimes, an inexperienced nurse isn't carefully screened before she's put on the job. Then, her lack of knowledge could lead to dangerous medication errors.

In one case, amazing as it sounds, a newly hired nurse administering lactulose didn't understand basic information about this drug, which is used in hepatic coma. One evening, when she went into the patient's room and found him unconscious, she returned the drug to the patient's bin rather than administer it through his tube. The reason she noted on the medication administration record was that he was sleeping!

Apparently, the nurse hadn't read any information about the drug even though she wasn't familiar with it.

Of course, the nurse should have at least gone to another nurse or pharmacist for clarification before she administered the dose. But a nurse who makes such a basic mistake usually doesn't know she's in error. So, new employees must be carefully screened and tested by the inservice coordinator or head nurse.

Notes:

_____

_____

_____

_____

_____

Neglecting to find out what's behind a patient's refusal to take medication

A patient's refusal to take his medicine can sometimes be considered a medication error because the refusal may be a result of improper patient education. This happened at one hospital where an alcoholic patient was admitted with delirium tremens. His doctor prescribed paraldehyde, and, since the patient was unruly, the doctor decided to have the drug administered orally. So the nurse mixed the paraldehyde with orange juice in a plastic cup with a plastic spoon—not realizing that paraldehyde dissolves many plastics. As the patient was about to drink his medicine, he noticed that the cup and spoon were melting. He threw the cup down and shouted, "I'm not taking that stuff—you're trying to kill me."

In this case, as in many cases of patient refusal, the understandable reluctance of the patient could have been avoided if the personnel had given the matter a little forethought.

Along with the indications, any aspect of his medication the patient may interpret as dangerous should be avoided or explained beforehand, whenever possible. Patients also need reassurance about unpleasant side effects of a medication. Usually, a patient will be more apt to take his medicine as prescribed when he is told how it will benefit him.

Notes:

Error
Number

146

Using the abbreviation "q.n." instead of "h.s." or the word "nightly"

When a doctor wrote the order below:

MOM 30 ml PO qn

he used the abbreviation "q.n." to mean "every night." Unfortunately, the administering nurse thought the order said "q.h" (every hour). After the patient developed severe diarrhea from hourly doses of milk of magnesia, the nurse realized the error.

The abbreviation "q.n." was not on the hospital's approved list. So the doctor should have used the standard "h.s." (at bedtime) or written the word "nightly" on his order.

But he didn't. Help to avoid these errors by getting serious about unauthorized, unfamiliar abbreviations when you realize that one has been used. Some of these abbreviations are dangerous and have been purposely left off your hospital's JCAHO approved list. Your patient's safety comes before anything else.

Notes:
_____

_____

_____

_____

_____

Not labeling I.V. bags when adding medications to them

At the start of a code, a nurse undid the sterile wrapper on a D_5W bag and added four 400 mg ampules of Intropin (dopamine hydrochloride). She put the bag on the crash cart next to the empty wrapper but didn't label the bag to show that the drug had been added. The I.V. was never started, though.

When the confusion of the code dissipated, another nurse saw the unused, unlabeled bag. Assuming it had just been taken from a nearby wrapper, she put it back into the wrapper and returned the package to the nurses' stock shelf.

About 20 minutes later, a third nurse entered the stockroom to pick up a D_5W bag for one of her patients. When she saw the opened package on the stock shelf, she assumed it'd been opened by mistake and contained a fresh bag. So she used it to start her patient's I.V.

Meanwhile, the first nurse was finishing her report on the code. Suddenly, she remembered the I.V. bag she'd mixed but hadn't hung. Fortunately, she located the bag before the third nurse's patient had received any of the solution.

In this instance, the patient escaped harm. But the consequences of this error could have been serious. So hang only I.V. bags you've unwrapped yourself—unless they were prepared and labeled in the pharmacy. And if you must add medication, be sure to label the bag immediately. For dopamine, you can completely avoid making infusion solutions if your hospital will purchase the premixed variety.

Notes:

_____

_____

_____

_____

_____

Error
Number

148

Relying on outdated PDRs or other old drug handbooks

A nurse received a doctor's order for Noroxin, 1 tablet b.i.d. But she wound up scheduling levothyroxine instead of norfloxacin. What happened?

Since the nurse wasn't familiar with Noroxin, she consulted an old drug handbook kept on the nursing unit. She couldn't find Noroxin in the book, but she did find Noroxine. Discounting the small spelling difference, she listed levothyroxine on the medication administration record.

She sent a copy of the order to the pharmacy. The pharmacist sent Noroxin. That's when she realized her error.

A similarity in drug names, and a nurse's false assumption, contributed to this medication error. Because Noroxin is a fairly new drug, it wasn't listed in this old drug reference. Noroxine, on the other hand, has undergone a name change, but it's still listed in some older reference books. Who knows what similar error will happen in the future—besides having similar names, some drug's usual doses even overlap.

To avoid such errors in your hospital, replace all your old drug reference books with the newest editions. Unless it's an extreme emergency, always have the pharmacist review the original order before giving the first dose.

Notes:

Not charting medication doses immediately after administering them

A student nurse was instructed to administer medication to her assigned patient. Since the patient was to receive a dose of indomethacin (Indocin) at 10 a.m. and another at 2 p.m., the pharmacist had put two prepackaged doses in the unit-dose medication cart. At 10 a.m., the student took the patient's medication administration record (MAR) from the MAR book, took one dose from the patient's drawer in the medication cart, administered the drug, and initialed the MAR. She kept it with her to chart the afternoon dose.

Meanwhile, the medication nurse arrived to give the patient his 10 a.m. dose. She checked the MAR book and found his MAR was missing. But instead of looking for it, she recalled the patient's order from the day before, pulled the remaining dose from his drawer in the cart, and administered it.

When the student nurse reported off the floor that afternoon, she returned the patient's MAR to the medication nurse, who then discovered the double dose.

This error happened because the medication nurse deviated from established charting practice. When she found the patient's MAR missing, she should have investigated further.

She also broke the cardinal rule for administering medication: Check the medication against the orders on the MAR when pulling the medication from the cart. Check it again when you're preparing to administer it. And check it once again when you've completed administration. Then initial the chart *immediately*.

Failure to chart doses immediately after administering them is one of the most common causes of medication errors. The error usually happens when someone other than the medication nurse is responsible for administering medications on the unit (e.g., students, doctors).

But charting doses before or long after they're administered can cause errors, too. For instance, if a nurse prerecords her initials, then rushes off to answer a code, chances are the patient won't get that dose. Or if she administers a drug intending to chart it later, another person can easily assume the dose wasn't given, and the patient will get a double dose.

So make charting medications a ritual: Initial the patient's MAR when you administer the medication.

Failing to assess medication orders routinely

A patient admitted for surgery brought with him some medications he'd been taking at home. Among them was a bottle of digoxin, containing tablets of 0.25 mg but labeled 2.5 mg. When the admitting doctor read the label, he wrote a pharmacy order for digoxin, 2.5 mg daily, without questioning the unusually high dose. Further, since the patient was to have nothing by mouth the day of surgery, the doctor ordered that day's dose to be given by injection.

Since the hospital used a partial floor-stock system, the nurse received a copy of the order and due to her inexperience did not suspect the order was in error. She administered the first dose before the hospital pharmacist could review it. When the pharmacist finally received the digoxin order along with the patient's medications from home, he immediately realized the dose was much too high. He checked the patient's bottle, saw that it was mislabeled, and realized what had happened.

The pharmacist called the nurse's station to report the error but was told the patient had already received his daily dose of digoxin by injection and had gone to surgery.

How many individual mistakes contributed to this medication error? First, the neighborhood pharmacist mislabeled the patient's digoxin bottle. Second, the admitting doctor took a shortcut and copied the order from the mislabeled bottle, rather than from the patient's prescription records. He compounded his mistake by failing to question the unusually high dose of a common drug and he changed the administration route without reducing the dose. These mistakes caused a toxic dose to be administered.

Third, the nurse giving the drug didn't assess the order—if she had, she'd have known the dose was too high. And since the hospital used some drugs from floor-stock, the hospital pharmacist didn't review the doctor's order until after the first dose was given.

This medication error occurred because the hospital's system of checks and balances broke down. To maintain that system methodically assess every medication order:
• when you first receive the order, to confirm that it makes sense
• when you obtain the medication
• when you prepare it for administration
• when you give it to the patient.

Additionally, make certain that you know the purpose of the drug, its dose, its contraindications, and its nursing implications.

Not confirming a patient's identity

A nurse administered 300 mg of allopurinol (Zyloprim) to Mr. Jones in room 205—or so she thought. Actually, Mr. Jones had been transferred out of room 205 and Mr. Smith moved in...without the nurse's knowledge. When questioned later, the nurse admitted she hadn't checked the patient's identification (ID) band because she'd given Mr. Jones his medication for several days and was sure she recognized him.

In a similar incident, a nurse gave Mrs. Paterson in room 815 the furosemide (frusemide, Lasix) and Robitussin intended for Mrs. Rossman—who was in the room's other bed. How did the nurse confuse the two patients?

Mrs. Rossman had just been admitted and wasn't in her assigned bed. Mrs. Paterson, who'd just been brought back to the room after undergoing a lab test, was mistakenly put in the wrong bed. She wasn't wearing her ID band because it had been removed during the test. So while the nurse thought she'd confirmed the patient's identity, she'd only confirmed the right bed.

In another case, a nurse approached the patient in bed A of room 711 and saw that he had no ID band. So she called out, "Mr. Stankowicz?"—the name on her medication order. The patient answered "yes," so she gave him the medications. Unfortunately, he was Mr. McCoy. Mr. Stankowicz was in the other bed.

Mr. McCoy probably had poor hearing or was heavily sedated, or possibly was suffering from organic brain syndrome. He may have thought he was helping the nurse by answering yes.

In another similar example, the nurse knew that one of the patients in room 252 was to have milk of magnesia. Since the patient in bed A didn't have an ID band, she asked him his last name. His answer, Williams, matched the name on her order, so she administered the milk of magnesia. Later, she discovered the order was for the patient in the other bed. His last name? Williams.

In all these cases where medication was given to the wrong patient, the error could have been avoided by confirming the patient's identity first. So always check the patient's ID band against your order sheet. If he's not wearing an ID band, ask the patient his name...first and last. Then confirm it with another nurse. And before you continue your rounds, get the patient a new ID band.

Error
Number

152

Being misled by unclear symbols

The U.S. Drug Enforcement Administration uses the symbols I, II, III, IV, and V to denote five classes of potentially dangerous drugs. In the United States, you'll see the symbol for any classified drug on its product label. But the class IV symbol, written Ⓘᵥ, is a potential trap for the unwary health professional. Here's how one nurse misinterpreted it:

A nurse who had been out of practice for nearly 20 years returned to work on a medical/surgical unit. This nurse received and transcribed an order for 10 mg of diazepam (Valium), to be given I.V. When she saw Ⓘᵥ on the box of diazepam tablets, she thought this signified hypodermic tablets that could be dissolved and given intravenously (hypodermic tablets were used 20 years ago). Then she compounded this error with poor sterile technique. She crushed a tablet in a mortar, added sterile water, drew up the dose in a syringe, and injected the solution into a patient.

When the error was discovered, the nurse explained she often prepared injectables from hypodermic tablets on her last job.

Another controlled drug that has been given intravenously instead of by its intended oral route is paraldehyde. Also, promethazine with Codeine Ⓥ, a class V substance, has been confused with promethazine VC.

To avoid this medication error, all new employees, whether graduates or experienced nurses, should be instructed to recognize this potentially misleading symbol.

Notes:

_____

_____

_____

_____

_____

Leaving medications meant for one patient within the reach of another

A patient took warfarin 20 mg, oxtriphylline 100 mg, and chlor-diazepoxide 10 mg that was meant for his roommate. How? When the medication nurse entered the room on her rounds, she found that the patient for whom the medications were intended was slipping out of bed. She hurriedly put the medicine on the closest clear surface—the nightstand of the other patient. Since he was accustomed to finding his own medications placed there, he took them while the nurse was busy.

Be aware that you might be interrupted when administering medications. Be ready to put the medications in a safe place until you can return to them. The best rule is: Never leave medications meant for one patient within the reach of another.

Notes:

Error
Number

154

Assuming that one package of medication equals one dose

A nurse administered furosemide (fruscmide, Lasix) 400 mg to a patient instead of 40 mg. The medication error resulted from the compounding of many smaller errors. The nurse that administered the medication had worked in a patient care area where the full unit-dose system was used. She was transferred to an area where the traditional dosage system was used. When she received an order for Lasix 40 mg, she found that the stock supply was depleted, so she called the pharmacy and ordered one dose of Lasix 40 mg. The pharmacist, to be helpful, sent her 10 tablets of Lasix, 40 mg per tablet, as a temporary supply. He put them all in a vial labeled, "Lasix 40 mg." The nurse, who was accustomed to the concept that one package equals one dose, administered the 10 tablets.

Insist that pharmacists label drugs as specifically as possible, particularly in hospitals that partially use the unit-dose system. When you have any doubt at all about a label, question it. This error would probably have been avoided if the pharmacist had labeled the drug properly, as shown: *furosemide (Lasix) 40 mg per tablet 10 tablets.*

Notes: _____

_____

_____

_____

_____

Administering Lugol's solution into an eye

The following order was written for a patient in preparation for administration of radioactive iodine (^{131}I):

Lugol's soln gtts x̄ OS q id

During rounds the next morning, the doctor asked the patient how he was feeling. The patient replied: "Pretty good—except for those eyedrops you're giving me. They really hurt." Knowing that no eyedrops had been ordered, the doctor checked the medication administration record and discovered his order had been misinterpreted.

The patient should have been given Lugol's solution orally, 10 drops in orange juice. The nurse transcribing the order interpreted OJ as OD (right eye). On two shifts the patient was given the Lugol's solution in his right eye.

If the doctor had used standard abbreviations, or if he had specified the route of administration, or if the nurses had realized that Lugol's solution is not for ophthalmic use, the error could have been avoided.

Notes:

_____

_____

_____

_____

Error Number	
156	

Allowing unqualified personnel to administer drugs

When the stock of injectable vitamin B_{12} was exhausted on a hospital unit, someone on the nursing staff called the pharmacist. Until the new supply arrived, she asked, would it be all right to substitute two doses of vitamin B_6 for the prescribed B_{12}.

This actually happened. And although laughable, it points to a fact of life...that we sometimes have inexperienced and possibly unqualified persons involved in administering medications.

The best way to guard against serious errors in these situations is to make sure you have a drug distribution that encourages checking and double-checking. You should also encourage questioning. Don't laugh at people when they ask what seems like a silly question. You may discourage them from asking other important questions in the future.

Notes:

Failing to observe dose precautions of analgesics for patients recovering from anesthetics

When Mrs. Roberts, who'd had a general anesthetic for a hysterectomy, was returned to her room, she began complaining of pain. In the recovery room, her surgeon had ordered meperidene hydrochloride (Demerol) 75 mg intramuscularly every 4 hours, p.r.n., pain, so the nurse gave her the ordered dose. Soon Mrs. Roberts became acutely hypotensive. Her surgeon, checking her chart, discovered that fentanyl citrate/droperidol (Innovar) had been administered to Mrs. Roberts while she was in surgery.

As you know, when the combination analgesic/neuroleptic, Innovar, is given during surgery, subsequent doses of narcotic analgesic drugs should be reduced, in some cases to as low as one third the usual dose. This precaution is necessary to avoid potentiating Innovar's respiratory depressant and hypotensive actions. Usually, the precaution must be observed for 4 to 6 hours after administration of the Innovar.

This precaution, though well known, is sometimes ignored because the doctor ordering the drugs simply forgets it, doesn't think the precaution is necessary, or doesn't know that the patient has received Innovar. Still, since the nurse giving the drugs shares the responsibility, she should question such orders.

Complications like those in Mrs. Roberts' case can be avoided by always following this procedure:
1. When the patient is given Innovar, the person administering the drug should immediately affix the label (which is coated with a reusable adhesive and comes as part of the drug package) to the metal front of the patient's chart.
2. The doctor ordering the Innovar should note on the label the period for which the precautions are in effect. If a narcotic analgesic is ordered later, this order should observe the reduction in dose for the time period.
3. When the patient and chart arrive on the nursing floor, the nurse or ward clerk noting the orders should peel the Innovar label off the chart and reaffix it directly on the patient's medication administration record. Also, the order as written by the doctor should be noted.

This procedure provides double insurance that the precautions will be followed—the initial order shows the reduced dosage and the sticker is a highly visible reminder.

Error
Number

158

Not knowing the patient's diagnosis or allergies

An oncologist instructed a medical student to write an order for 8 mg daily of chlorambucil (Leukeran) on the chart of a patient with Hodgkin's disease. The student inadvertently wrote the order on the chart of the patient's roommate (who had been admitted for an appendectomy). The order was processed by the nursing and pharmacy personnel and the drug was given to the wrong patient for 2 weeks. The mistake was discovered only when a routine blood count showed the patient receiving the drug had a severe bone marrow depression.

Probably, your first reaction is to blame the medication error directly on the student. Actually, the responsibility must also be shouldered by others.

First, the oncologist disobeyed the hospital's rule that all orders written by students must be countersigned by a doctor. Second, the pharmacists and nurses should not have carried out an order that wasn't properly countersigned. Third, and most important, the nurses and pharmacists should have known the diagnosis of the patient for whom the order was written.

Giving drugs, particularly cancer drugs, is a tremendous responsibility. Those administering the drugs must know the patient's diagnosis as well as his allergies—if any—and make sure these are noted on the patient profile and Kardex.

All this seems so basic that many of us assume it's automatically done. Yet, far too often, when the people administering the drugs are asked if they've checked out the patient's diagnosis or allergies, they answer, "I didn't have the time," or "It just slipped my mind." Obviously, these answers wouldn't hold up in court, if litigation resulted from a medication error. And, bringing it closer to home, if your loved one were injured by a medication error, how would *you* react to such an explanation?

Notes:

Forgetting to check with your unit clerk on new orders

159

On a busy CCU, nurses on walking rounds discovered a patient on a D_5W I.V., TKO. (This was a standing order on the unit, to maintain an open line to a patient's circulatory system.)

But the patient's Kardex called for something else: 5% dextrose in ½ normal saline solution at 50 ml/hour. During the previous shift, the patient had become mildly dehydrated, so the doctor had written new orders. By the time the nurses discovered the new charted orders, several hours had passed.

What had gone wrong? On this unit, the unit clerk was supposed to note the doctor's orders on the Kardex and relay this information to the nurses. But the above order wasn't an emergency, and the unit clerk had forgotten to notify nurses on the previous shift about the changed order.

As a nurse, what can you do to help the unit clerk keep you informed? You could suggest that she use a flagging system that doesn't rely on memory. For example, the unit clerk could place a paper clip on a patient's Kardex as she tears off the order copy destined for pharmacy.

Even so, don't assume the unit clerk will always follow the system. If you're working on a small unit like CCU, try to make rounds with the doctor, so you know what he's writing on the patients' charts. If you're on a larger unit, and you see the doctor on the floor, check with the unit clerk automatically about any new orders.

Notes:

_____

_____

_____

_____

_____

Error
Number

160

Neglecting to mix the contents of two vials

A doctor ordered a stat dose of I.V. glucagon, 1 mg, for a diabetic patient who was having a hypoglycemic reaction. The nurse was to give a second 1-mg dose in 20 minutes if he didn't respond. The order was given at change of shift, so two nurses administered the doses.

The pharmacist had dispensed two boxes of glucagon, each containing a 1-mg vial of lyophilized glucagon powder for injection and a 1-ml vial of diluent. The next day, when he was preparing the unit-dose cassettes, he noticed that the patient's drawer still contained one vial of the powder. Because the diluent was gone, he suspected that one of the nurses had mistakenly administered just the diluent.

He was right. Although the vials were clearly labeled "Vial 1 (diluent for glucagon injection)" and "Vial 2 (glucagon for injection)," the nurse who prepared and administered one of the doses apparently hadn't read the labels carefully. She hadn't mixed the contents of the vials.

Of course, if she'd read the labels, she would have avoided this error. But the pharmacist could have helped out by putting a second label on each vial or on the carton containing the vials, reminding the nurse to mix the contents. Or he even could have mixed them himself before dispensing the drug.

Notes:

Not knowing that the abbreviation "5-ASA" stands for "5-aminosalicylic acid"

A new staff nurse was passing out medications for the first time. She was doing well until she came across an order for "5-ASA at bedtime." She opened a box of unit-dose aspirin and prepared to give the patient five aspirin tablets. The supervisor caught her in time and explained that the order was for mesalamine (Rowasa) enema, a relatively new drug used to treat ulcerative colitis.

For years, doctors treated ulcerative colitis with an oral drug, sulfasalazine (Azulfidine). The active metabolite of sulfasalazine is 5-aminosalicylic acid, or, as it's sometimes called, 5-ASA. Mesalamine is a formulation composed purely of that metabolite, and sometimes a doctor will improperly use the abbreviation 5-ASA when ordering the new drug.

The doctor wrote the order for 5-ASA, then compounded his error by giving an incomplete order. If he'd specified that mesalamine is an enema, or included directions, the new nurse might have questioned the order.

One way to reduce the chance that this mistake will occur is to discourage doctors from using 5-ASA as an abbreviation. Another is simply to be aware that the problem exists.

Notes:

_____

_____

_____

_____

Being unaware of look-alike Tubexes

Error
Number

162

A patient's heparin lock needed to be flushed because it was obstructed with blood. His nurse went to the medication room, reached into a bin marked "Hep-flush kits," and withdrew what she thought were Tubexes of saline solution and heparin.

She returned to the patient's room and injected the saline solution. As she withdrew the needle, she noted that the label on the Tubex read, "dimenhydrinate injection" instead of "sodium chloride injection." She'd administered a 50-mg dose of the generic equivalent of Dramamine. After notifying the doctor immediately, she closely monitored the patient, who slept soundly that day but suffered no other ill effects from the dimenhydrinate.

You know that you should read labels at least three times: when taking a dose from a patient's bin or the drug storage area, when preparing or administering the dose, and when discarding a drug container or *returning it to stock*. That last step can't be overemphasized. If you return a look-alike drug to the wrong storage area, someone else may bypass the first label check and pick up the wrong drug, which is exactly what happened here.

Notes:

Being careless when giving morphine to a child

A 19-month-old boy was admitted to the emergency department (ED) of a small community hospital after an automobile accident. He was screaming from the severe pain of a leg fracture, so the doctor ordered 2 mg of morphine liquid, to be given orally. Several hours later, the boy died from a morphine overdose. His autopsy revealed that he'd received approximately 20 times the ordered dose.

Although morphine solutions come in concentrations of 2 mg/ml and 4 mg/ml, this hospital had only Roxanol, 20 mg/ml, which is usually given to cancer patients. The cap on a Roxanol bottle has a calibrated dropper marked 1 ml, 1.5 ml, and 2 ml.

The ED nurse should have drawn up 0.1 ml of Roxanol, but that amount wasn't scored on the dropper. She may have measured 2 ml on the dropper, thinking it was 2 mg—the correct dose. Or, she may have drawn up 1 ml (20 mg), incorrectly interpreting it as 0.1 ml.

Administering morphine to a child requires extreme caution. Liquid doses are best prepared and labeled by pharmacists, using special oral syringes that won't accommodate a needle. Dose calculations and preparations should be checked by at least two people—ideally, a pharmacist and a nurse, who could also double-check their interpretations of the order. Concentrated morphine should be kept only in the pharmacy. It's too dangerous to be on the unit, where it may be misused.

Notes:

_____

_____

_____

_____

_____

<table>
<tr>
<td>

Error
Number

164

</td>
<td>

Not reporting diagnostic test results accurately

Mr. Ferguson and Mr. Redpath, two diabetic patients assigned to the same room, had orders for glucose tests to be followed by insulin administration as needed.

The nurse caring for these two patients was very busy, so she asked the nursing assistant to perform the tests. The assistant did so and gave the nurse values indicating that Mr. Ferguson didn't need insulin whereas Mr. Redpath did. The nurse administered insulin to Mr. Redpath, as ordered, then went to dinner.

Within a few minutes, the nurse was paged and asked to return to the unit immediately. When she got there, Mr. Redpath was being treated for hypoglycemia. The nurse quickly checked Mr. Redpath's glucose test sheet and saw that the assistant had charted his test result as 90 mg/100 ml—an amount not requiring insulin. She then checked Mr. Ferguson's test sheet and saw that his result had been charted with the value she'd been given for Mr. Redpath. At this point, the nurse realized that the assistant had misinformed her, and she'd given the insulin to the wrong patient.

After Mr. Redpath's condition had stabilized and Mr. Ferguson had been given the appropriate dose of insulin, the head nurse called the nurse and the assistant into her office. She told them they shared the responsibility for this error. Referring to the hospital's policy and procedure manual, the head nurse pointed out that the nurse who administered insulin is responsible for performing the tests that determine the need for insulin.

Although this is a good policy to follow, it may not be practical for all hospitals. The best way to avoid such an error is to be sure all information you convey is accurate.

</td>
</tr>
</table>

Notes:

_____

_____

_____

_____

_____

Forgetting to verify the quantity of drug per vial

Hospital employees should always read labels carefully before they prepare dosages. But they should be especially careful when new labels appear on familiar products. In one case, a nurse misinterpreted a poorly written label and gave a patient 10 times the dose of chloramphenicol sodium succinate (Chloromycetin Sodium Succinate) that the doctor prescribed.

The error began with a new, redesigned label (from the manufacturer) on a vial of chloramphenicol. The old label had stated clearly that the vial contained 1 g of chloramphenicol. But then the new label was substituted—a label that didn't state the quantity of drug per vial. Instead, it stated that 1 ml of the reconstituted drug would contain 100 mg of chloramphenicol.

A nurse who needed 2 g of chloramphenicol glanced at the new label and thought the *entire vial* contained only 100 mg of chloramphenicol. So she reconstituted 20 1-g vials and injected the drug. The patient died 11 hours later.

Poor labeling on the vial cannot be blamed entirely for this medication error. How could someone responsible for administering drugs reconstitute and inject 20 vials of a drug without thinking that something was wrong? How could someone administer a drug without knowing anything about its side effects and toxicity?

Clearly, this should never have happened. Yet in 1975, it actually did. At least five patients were accidentally given ten times the intended dose of chloramphenicol, according to a letter in the *Journal of the American Medical Association* (October 13, 1975). As a result, the manufacturer redesigned the label, clarifying the contents. Still we occasionally receive similar reports involving other drugs.

So if, for any reason, you ever find yourself in a position of needing to administer any dosage of more than one or two units (capsules, tablets, vials, or ampules), check with another nurse or a pharmacist.

Notes:

Error Number

166

Giving "Mustargen" instead of "methotrexate"

A pharmacist working in a pharmacy-run Injection Preparation Service received an order for "MTX 30 mg I.M. now." For some reason, even though he knew better, he thought of Mustargen as being the same as methotrexate. The abbreviation MTX signifies methotrexate. He reconstituted three 10 mg vials with one milliliter of sterile water for each vial and prepared a syringe containing 30 mg of Mustargen in 3 ml, thinking that this was actually methotrexate. The drug was to be administered to a psoriasis patient on a dermatology patient care area where methotrexate injection was commonly used. The pharmacist handed the syringe to a nurse and mentioned to her that for some reason he just didn't think everything seemed right. He was leery about administering the drug intramuscularly. The nurse assured him that methotrexate was given intramuscularly frequently and that everything was all right. But when the nurse looked at the pharmacy-prepared and -labeled syringe, she was surprised to see a different color and volume than she was used to seeing. However, since the syringe was properly labeled and was prepared by a pharmacist, she assumed that everything was correct and administered the drug in the patient's buttock.

Approximately two hours later, the patient began complaining of buttock pain. The nurse then became suspicious and called the pharmacist and it was then realized that Mustargen was administered—not methotrexate.

Immediate attempts were made to find information about how the effects of this necrotizing agent could be reversed. A one-sixth molar solution of sodium thiosulfate (prepared as described in the Mustargen package insert) was infiltrated in 5 ml doses in five spaces around the area of injection. No other therapy was discovered. Even the manufacturer of Mustargen was unable to be of help.

Contrary to what was expected, the patient miraculously suffered no toxicity from the dose or from the local effects as long as one month later.

Several things need to be examined about this incident in order to prevent similar errors in the future.

First of all, the abbreviation MTX should not have been used. This is initially what made the pharmacist think of Mustargen. Medications must always be prescribed by their official name.

Secondly, if the pharmacist was thinking that something didn't seem right, he should have had a colleague check the work he was doing. An examination of the vials used (Mustargen) by another pharmacist would have prevented the error.

Finally, the nurse who received the syringed and labeled medication from the pharmacist put blind faith in the pharmacist's work. The nurse recognized that a different color and volume of liquid than she was used to seeing with methotrexate injection was present in the syringe. Yet she failed to question the pharmacist because she trusted his work. One of the advantages of unit-dose systems with prepared syringed injections is that a double-check exists before the patient receives the medication (pharmacist and nurse). This would not be true if the nurse prepared the injection. Errors in volume for the particular drug or route of administration are more easily discovered with a double-check, and color differences may be questioned to learn if the wrong drug was prepared. But you must question any recognized discrepancies.

Notes:

Being careless with neuromuscular blockers

After developing severe respiratory problems, a 79-year-old woman was intubated and placed on a ventilator. She was tachycardic and restless; her respirations were 48.

The intensive care unit (ICU) nurse who was suctioning her met with some resistance, but she continued the procedure and told another nurse that everything was fine. Soon, the ventilator alarms went off, indicating that the patient was bucking the ventilator or otherwise exerting negative pressure.

The nurse immediately called the doctor, who ordered I.V. morphine, 10 mg, to relax her. When that didn't work, she called him again and he ordered pancuronium bromide (Pavulon), a neuromuscular blocker that paralyzes restless patients and allows the ventilator to take over respirations.

Minutes after the drug was administered, the patient's respirations stopped and her heart rate dropped to 30. Manual bagging didn't help, although atropine did restore her heart rate. After vigorous suctioning, the nurse removed a large mucus plug. Ventilation was resumed, but the patient died several days later.

In another case, a doctor ordered Pavulon for a ventilator patient, to be given "p.r.n. for agitation." The patient was doing well and began breathing on his own, so he no longer needed the ventilator.

After a family visit, though, he became flustered and seemed so disturbed that a new ICU nurse checked the medication administration record to see if his doctor had written an order for an antianxiety drug. She saw that Pavulon had been ordered for agitation. Although unfamiliar with Pavulon, she took the drug from the medication cabinet and administered it. Immediately, the patient went into respiratory arrest. A code was called and he was resuscitated, but not before permanent brain damage.

Both examples show that neuromuscular blocking agents like Pavulon require specific protocols that include the following cautions:
• The patient must be on a ventilator.
• Only an anesthesiologist or a critical care nurse who's educated about the drug and who's administered it before should give an ordered neuromuscular blocker.
• The drug shouldn't be administered until the patient has a patent airway.
• The order for the drug must be automatically discontinued when the patient is removed from the ventilator.
• A doctor's order should never say "p.r.n. for agitation."

Confusing "Percocet" with "Percocet-5"

A patient's medication administration record read, "Percocet-5 every 3 to 4 hours as needed for pain." Twice, over the next 24 hours, a nurse administered *five* tablets each from a bottle marked "Percocet."

What the doctor had meant was *one* tablet per dose of a drug formerly called Percocet-5. Luckily, the patient was only oversedated; he didn't experience a more serious adverse reaction.

Percocet (oxycodone), an oral analgesic, was called Percocet-5 until a few years ago, when the manufacturer dropped the 5. Now the label reads "Percocet"—exactly what these nurses saw when they went into the unit's narcotics cabinet.

Some health professionals, like this doctor, still call the drug Percocet-5. If your hospital stocks Percocet, be on the lookout for confusion over the name. You might ask the pharmacist to place a second label on the box to alert nurses to the drug's former name.

Notes:

Error
Number

169

Ordering a central venous line prematurely

A staff nurse was helping an I.V. team nurse flush a multilumen central venous catheter. The catheter had been inserted 3 days earlier because the doctor wanted to start the patient on total parenteral nutrition (TPN), but he hadn't ordered it yet.

According to hospital procedure, the I.V. nurse was supposed to flush each port of the catheter with 10 ml of normal saline solution, followed by 1.5 to 2 ml of heparin flush solution, 100 units/ml. The staff nurse mistakenly picked up a vial of heparin, *10,000* units/ml. Without checking the label, she prepared the heparin flush solutions to be used at the three ports. The patient received 60,000 units of heparin and later began bleeding from his nose, urinary tract, and bowel.

Obviously, if either nurse had read the heparin label, this serious error could have been prevented. But we should consider other factors. Why did the nurse even have to draw up the heparin? Several manufacturers package heparin flush solutions in syringes in various strengths. The nurse need only have reached for three ready-to-use syringes.

Also, why was heparin available in the unit's stock at 10,000 units/ml? That concentration should be issued by the pharmacy only for specific patients.

Finally, why was a central venous line in place if it wasn't being used? If it hadn't been ordered prematurely, the error would never have occurred.

Notes:
_____
_____
_____
_____
_____

Giving a drug without checking the MAR

A few minutes before afternoon report, the day medication nurse gave a patient 7.5 mg of warfarin (Coumadin), then charted what she'd done in the medication administration record (MAR). When the evening medication nurse asked the nurse giving report if the patient had received the drug, she said she didn't know.

After report, the evening medication nurse took a dose of Coumadin into the patient's room and asked him if he'd been given the drug. The patient said he'd received a new medication about an hour earlier, but he didn't know its name. The nurse left the Coumadin on the patient's bedside stand and went to check the MAR. She discovered that the patient had received the Coumadin, so she went to retrieve the drug from the patient's room. But the patient had already taken it.

What went wrong? First, the evening medication nurse shouldn't have tried to give the drug without checking the MAR before she went into the patient's room. Second, she shouldn't have left medication on the bedside stand. Finally, if the day medication nurse had educated the patient about his new drug, he could have told the other nurse what he'd taken.

Notes:

_____

_____

_____

_____

Error
Number

171

Borrowing a dose from another patient's supply or from stock on the nursing unit

A 75-year-old postmastectomy patient had a history of congestive heart failure. When her condition began to worsen, her doctor ordered 40 mg of furosemide (frusemide, Lasix) stat. Her nurse had another patient receiving 40 mg of Lasix, so she borrowed a dose and gave it to the postmastectomy patient. Later, the nurse transcribed the order and sent it to the pharmacy. The pharmacist immediately telephoned the unit and told the nurse to withhold the Lasix because the patient was allergic to the drug.

In her haste, the nurse hadn't checked the patient's medication administration record or chart. After the call from the pharmacist, she went back to the patient's room and discovered that the patient had already developed a rash on her trunk and face. The nurse called the doctor and got an order for diphenhydramine (Benadryl) to counteract the patient's adverse reaction.

Unless a true emergency exists, don't let a doctor's request for stat medication interfere with your responsibility to check your patient's records for allergies or other contraindications. If you borrow a dose from another patient's supply or from stock on the nursing unit, you're bypassing the safety net that the hospital has set up to prevent errors like this one—the nurse-pharmacist double-check.

Notes:

Confusing Roman numeral four (IV) with intravenous (I.V.)

A doctor whose patient was going through alcohol withdrawal called in an order for 5 ml of paraldehyde. He wanted it to be given orally, but his order was incomplete—he didn't specify the administration route.

A nurse who was unfamiliar with the drug took a container of paraldehyde from the floor stock. She saw C_{IV} printed on the label. Assuming that meant she could administer the drug intravenously, she began drawing up the dose into a syringe. Another nurse saw what she was doing and stopped her.

Paraldehyde is classified as a Schedule IV drug under the Controlled Substances Act. The "IV" in the symbol C_{IV} on its containers stands for the Roman numeral four, not "intravenous."

Until recently, paraldehyde was available in sterile containers and could be given orally, rectally, or parenterally. For economic reasons, the manufacturer stopped making the sterile form. Some health professionals, unfamiliar with this change, may believe it still exists. But currently no injectable form is being manufactured.

Unless the U.S. Drug Enforcement Administration changes the symbol, an error like this will happen again. In fact, diazepam, phenobarbital, and chloral hydrate—also drugs in the C_{IV} category—all have been erroneously administered I.V.

Notes:

Error
Number

173

Not returning vials to their storage bins

A nurse working in a busy outpatient clinic was preparing an I.V. dose of the antiemetic dexamethasone (Decadron) for a man receiving cancer chemotherapy. She took a multidose vial of Decadron from a storage bin and set it on the cluttered work table. After double-checking the label, she turned to get a syringe and needle, then picked up the vial and withdrew the dose. She gave the drug and the patient went home.

A short time later, the nurse noticed an unused vial of Decadron and a partially used vial of heparin on the work table. She realized at once what she'd done: She'd given the patient I.V. heparin instead of Decadron. Calculating quickly, she determined that she'd given him 25,000 units of heparin.

The nurse called the doctor, then the patient, who had to return to the clinic for a partial thromboplastin time (PTT). Although the patient's PTT was elevated, he didn't need treatment and was sent home with instructions to avoid taking aspirin and to report any signs of bleeding.

This incident could have been prevented if the heparin vial had been returned to the storage bin—either by the nurse who took it out or by the nurse preparing the Decadron. Keep drug areas free of clutter. Prepare one drug at a time, and dispose of used containers properly. And *always* read the label on a drug vial immediately before you draw the dose into the syringe.

Notes: _____

_____

_____

_____

Failing to confirm unusually high blood glucose levels

A 40-year-old woman was taken to a hospital emergency department (ED) suffering from gastrointestinal bleeding, nausea, and weakness. A nurse started an infusion of 5% dextrose in lactated Ringer's solution in the patient's right hand. Then she called the laboratory to send someone to draw samples for blood analysis.

A laboratory technician went to the ED, drew the blood, and returned to the laboratory to do the tests. Within minutes, she called the doctor to report a blood glucose level of 960 mg/dl.

The doctor immediately ordered the solution being infused changed to normal saline solution with 20 mEq of potassium chloride added. He also ordered a bolus of 10 units of regular insulin, followed by a second infusion containing regular insulin.

An hour later, the patient showed signs of hypoglycemia. Another blood sample was drawn; this time the glucose level was only 39 mg/dl. The doctor stopped the insulin infusion and gave 50% dextrose I.V. He also ordered the first infusion changed back to the original solution. Two hours later, the patient's glucose level was 90 mg/dl—within normal limits.

What happened? Simple—the laboratory technician had taken the first blood samples from a vein in the patient's right arm, the same arm being used for the dextrose infusion.

Don't let yourself be fooled by such an obvious mistake. Be suspicious when a blood glucose level is abnormally high, and confirm it before starting treatment.

Notes:

_____

_____

_____

_____

_____

Error
Number

175

Being misled by a number preceding a drug name

A doctor on evening rounds wrote this order for a leukemic patient:

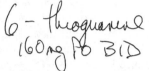

The nurse administering medications that evening wasn't familiar with this drug, but she didn't look it up. She thought about calling the hospital pharmacy, but it was closed for the night.

Anxious to start the patient's drug therapy and continue her rounds, the nurse decided to give the dose without checking it. She found a bottle labeled *thioguanine 40 mg,* left over from another patient, in the nursing unit's drug cabinet. Thinking that the "6" preceding the drug name on the doctor's order meant the number of doses, she calculated the amount as 960 mg (6 x 160 mg), and administered this dose to the patient. She then charted the dose she'd given as *thioguanine, 960 mg, P.O., tonight.*

The next morning on rounds, the doctor discovered the error. The patient, who'd complained of nausea and vomiting during the night, was later found to have severe bone marrow depression—a direct result of the overdose. Fortunately, he survived the incident, but overdoses of thioguanine have caused death.

The error could have been avoided if the doctor hadn't written the prefix "6," which is a remnant of the drug's chemical name. Most references to the drug, including the manufacturer's label, don't use this prefix. (Other drugs you may see written this way are 6 mercaptopurine, 5 fluorouracil, and 5 flucytosine.)

But the nurse could have prevented the error, too, by not giving the drug until she got more information about it. When she couldn't reach a pharmacist, she could have called her nursing supervisor or the doctor, or consulted a drug reference.

A change in hospital policy could have prevented this error, too: Routine orders for cancer chemotherapy should be initiated only when a pharmacist is available. Because these drugs are extremely toxic, a pharmacist should review the order and dispense the drug himself. The nurse should always check what the pharmacist dispenses against what the doctor's order specifies before she administers the drug.

Agreeing to leave medication with a patient when he asks

A doctor ordered chloral hydrate, 500 mg nightly, as a bedtime sedative for his patient. Each evening before ending her shift, the nurse brought the patient a capsule of chloral hydrate. Whenever the patient asked her to leave it on the nightstand so he could take it later, the nurse obliged.

After several days of hospitalization, the patient was sent to the X-ray department for studies. While the patient was off the floor, housekeeping personnel making his bed discovered eight capsules of chloral hydrate stuffed in a pillow. They reported their find to the head nurse. When the nurse asked the patient about the capsules, he admitted he'd been saving them for a suicide attempt.

To prevent any more such close calls, the hospital administration reinforced, in writing, its policy that nurses stay with patients while they take their medications.

Unfortunately, leaving oral medications on a patient's nightstand and not staying to see that he takes the drugs is too common a practice. Often the patient requests this...or he's out of the room during medication administration rounds. Although this practice *seems* harmless, it definitely increases the risk of medication error.

When more than one patient is in the room, for example, a patient may mistakenly take his roommate's medication. Or, as this case illustrates, he may not take his medication at all. In any case, the patient may not receive what his doctor ordered.

Certain medications, however, such as antacids, nitroglycerin, and some topical preparations, can be given to a patient to self-administer. And in some hospitals, certain patients participate in self-medication programs. But in either case, the hospital must have a policy stating the doctor writes the medication order.

If a patient asks you to leave his medication for him to take later, refuse, and try to convince him to take it right away. If he won't cooperate, say no to the request. For p.r.n. medications and bedtime sedatives, offer to come back later when the patient wants to take the dose. And above all, stay with the patient until you're sure he's swallowed the medication.

Error
Number

177

Confusing "Burroughs Wellcome" with "Burow's Solution"

A nurse took a telephone order from a doctor to irrigate a patient's bladder with sterile Neosporin G.U. Irrigant, an antibiotic solution manufactured by Burroughs Wellcome. When referring to the irrigant, however, the doctor incorrectly called it *Burroughs' solution*.

The nurse assumed the doctor meant *Burow's* solution, a topical astringent. So she wrote on the patient's chart: Irrigate bladder b.i.d., via catheter, with Burow's solution. The patient received several irrigations with Burow's solution.

The doctor found the error when he countersigned the order. Fortunately, the patient suffered no ill effects from irrigation with the nonsterile astringent...but he didn't receive the antibiotic's intended benefits, either.

From this experience, the nurse, doctor, and pharmacist learned firsthand about the danger of telephone orders—what's heard isn't always what's being requested. To prevent this confusion, always question the doctor when you're not familiar with a drug's name. Then, when checking with the pharmacist, tell him exactly why the drug's being prescribed.

Finally, work toward establishing a policy that doctors countersign telephone orders within 24 hours...and that those orders be limited to emergencies.

Notes:

Mistaking "folinic acid" for "folic acid"

A cancer patient was scheduled to receive a course of methotrex-ate therapy, followed 6 hours later by a dose of leucovorin cal-cium (folinic acid). In this procedure, known as rescue therapy, leucovorin calcium counteracts some of methotrexate's adverse systemic effects. The doctor wrote the order as folinic acid.

When the medication nurse took the leucovorin calcium to the patient 6 hours after the methotrexate course was completed, he fell asleep. The nurse confused folinic acid with folic acid, a vi-tamin. Thinking she wouldn't wake him for "just a vitamin," she withheld the dose. It was administered the next morning. Fortu-nately, the patient suffered no ill effects.

Certainly, the medication nurse who was unfamiliar with the official name for folinic acid erred in her judgment to withhold the dose without consulting the doctor. But other safeguards could have prevented this error. For another thing, the pharma-cist could have attached a label explaining leucovorin calcium's action in methotrexate therapy. For another, the doctor could have written the official generic name, leucovorin calcium, on the order to avoid confusion.

But the best way to prevent this error would have been to make sure all staff members who handle drugs understand them thoroughly. If the nurse had known why the folinic acid was to be administered, she wouldn't have assumed it was "just a vita-min."

Notes:
_____
_____
_____
_____
_____

Error
Number

179

Confusing "Librium" with "lithium"

A young man was admitted to a medical/surgical unit for treatment of severe depression. The psychiatrist initiated antidepressant therapy with amitriptyline (Elavil).

The next day, after a session with the psychiatrist, the patient became anxious and angry and began breaking furniture in his room. To control the patient's anxiety, the psychiatrist wrote a stat order for Librium (chlordiazepoxide), 100 mg, P.O.

The unit clerk misinterpreted the doctor's handwriting and transcribed the order as *lithium*, 100 mg, P.O., stat. The medication nurse who checked the order also interpreted the doctor's order as lithium. Then, because the order was stat, she borrowed a lithium tablet (available only in 300-mg strength) from another patient's supply. She divided the tablet into thirds and gave the patient one portion.

Since lithium has no calming effect on this type of behavior, the patient's anxiety didn't subside. The nurse called the psychiatrist to report that the patient's behavior hadn't changed. He immediately gave a stat verbal order for Librium, 50 mg, I.M.—assuming the first dose hadn't achieved the desired effect. When the nurse heard the psychiatrist say *Librium,* she realized the two drug names had been confused and that an error had been made.

Fortunately, the patient suffered no ill effects from the lithium, and the Librium injection did quell his anxiety.

Several actions (or lack of actions) added up to this medication error. Unquestionably, the psychiatrist's handwriting was not clear. But consider these points:
• The pharmacy was bypassed when the nurse borrowed a tablet from another patient's supply rather than send the order to the pharmacy. As a result, a pharmacist, who probably would have dispensed the correct drug, didn't see the order.
• The nurse didn't know that lithium isn't a stat drug. Since she wasn't familiar with the drug, she should have looked it up. Then she probably would have questioned the choice of drug.
• The nurse had to divide the tablet into thirds to administer the dose ordered. Because one third of a tablet is such an unusual dose, she should have suspected something was amiss.

Being careless when administering narcotics to postoperative patients

A doctor wrote the following order for a postoperative patient:

[handwritten order: Meperidine 25 mg IM until 4 pm then 50 mg IM prn q3h for pain]

Attached to the patient's chart was a sticker saying he'd received the anesthetic Innovar before his surgery.

At 3 p.m., the patient complained of pain. The medication nurse checked his medication administration record, obtained what she thought was the correct analgesic from the unit-dose narcotic floor stock, and administered it.

Moments later, the charge nurse checked the meperidine control form and noticed the medication nurse hadn't signed out any doses. When questioned, the medication nurse insisted she'd signed the form. When she produced the form, the charge nurse saw it was for *morphine*. The medication nurse had mistakenly read morphine for meperidine.

The usual dose of morphine is 10 to 12 mg. But when the patient has received Innovar, the morphine should be reduced to 4 mg. This is because the patient still had some anesthetic in his blood, and certain anesthetics, including Innovar, contain narcotics. So if the narcotic analgesic dose isn't reduced, this dose on top of the anesthetic's narcotic could be high enough to cause respiratory depression.

Since this patient had received about six times the safe dose of morphine, he developed respiratory distress and had to be given a narcotic antagonist to counteract the overdose.

This medication error could have been avoided if the medication nurse had carefully read the order. She also should have known a dose of 25 mg of morphine is too high for any patient. Further, she should have double-checked the dose when she saw the warning sticker on the patient's chart.

If you administer narcotics to postoperative patients, you should know about their dangerous additive effects on anesthetics. Always check to see what anesthetics a patient received, read all warning stickers, and question anything that seems out of order. Your extra caution could save a patient's life.

Using inaccurate measuring devices
for oral medications

A pediatrician ordered ampicillin suspension (125 mg/5 ml) 1 teaspoon, q.i.d., to be given to his patient for 10 days. The pharmacy dispensed the 10-day supply is a 200-ml bottle. Eight days after the child started receiving the antibiotic, a nursing instructor on a pediatric rotation noticed that the bottle was only half empty, when 80% of the medication should have been given. Yet all doses were signed for on the medication administration record.

The instructor asked the nurses how they were administering the antibiotic. They showed her the colorful plastic teaspoons they'd obtained from the dietary department to administer oral liquids to children. When the instructor measured a spoon's capacity, she found it to be less than 3 ml. The child hadn't received his proper dose of 5 ml at any time during the 8 days.

The volumes of different teaspoons may vary by up to 100%, and even medication cups aren't always accurate. So make sure your drug administration equipment includes accurate measuring devices for oral liquids, or better yet, try to get the pharmacy to dispense medications in unit-dose form.

One idea might be to use a 5-ml syringe to administer a teaspoon of medication. But this practice could be more dangerous than an inaccurate measurement; someone could mistakenly attach a needle and inject the suspension.

A better idea would be to use a specially designed syringe that won't accommodate a needle. Ask your pharmacist to package liquid doses this way for children or about ordering these syringes for your unit. But be careful; even these devices have been used for injection when placed on the Luer-Lok receptor of an indwelling intravenous catheter.

One final note: Warn patients taking oral liquids at home about the volume variances of different teaspoons. Supply them with accurate measuring devices if they're available.

Notes:

Not double-checking medication orders that are crossed out

A doctor ordered gentamicin, 60 mg, I.M., q14h, to control a *Pseudomonas* infection in a patient who had severe renal impairment. He wrote the unusual dosage because gentamicin is especially dangerous for patients with renal disease unless it's given according to a specific calculated formula. When he double-checked his calculations, though, he realized the order should have been q24h. But instead of crossing out the first order and rewriting it, he just wrote a "2" over the "1" in "14", so it looked like this:

When the nurse read the medication order, she thought the "2" had been crossed out and interpreted the order as q4h. She administered the first dose. Luckily, the charge nurse noticed the crossed-out number when she was reviewing the medication Kardex and checked it with the doctor. When she learned what he intended to order and compared that with what the nurse had given, she corrected the misinterpreted order before any more doses were given.

The highest recommended daily dose of gentamicin for patients with *normal* renal function is usually 5 mg/kg. So the nurse should have questioned a total daily dose of 360 mg for this 50 kg patient with renal disease.

Even if a doctor's written medication order is illegible, *you* can be held liable if you give the patient the wrong medication or dosage. So what should you do? Question anything on a medication order that could be interpreted more than one way. But the best way to protect a patient and yourself is to check the patient's diagnosis and the drugs prescribed to see if the order makes sense. And double-check anything crossed out on a medical order.

Error Number	Allowing stress to keep you from administering medication properly

183

A prisoner from a county jail was hospitalized for gallbladder surgery. During his first postoperative day, he developed a bad case of hiccups. His nurse tried several comfort measures to relieve the hiccups without success.

The patient soon became agitated by the constant tension on his suture line. His two guards also began to be concerned, and the three men bombarded the nurse with constant demands for relief of the hiccups.

Yielding to their pressure, the nurse called the patient's doctor, who ordered chlorpromazine (Thorazine), 50 mg I.M., stat. She quickly obtained the drug from floor stock and administered it, planning to chart the medication order afterward.

When the nurse checked the patient a short time later, he said, "That shot really helped. What was it anyway?"

"Thorazine," the nurse told him.

"Thorazine—I'm *allergic* to Thorazine!" yelled the patient.

The nurse checked his chart. Sure enough, both his chart and his medication administration record (MAR) had large stickers reading *Allergic to Thorazine*. Also, the patient was wearing a red hospital bracelet with the same warning.

The nurse immediately called the doctor, who told her to watch the patient closely. Fortunately, the patient, who'd had a dystonic reaction to Thorazine in the past, and not really an allergy, had no adverse reaction this time.

A tense situation caused this nurse to panic and skip a vital step in the medication administration process, which is: Check for allergies or a history of adverse reactions before administering a drug. She should have checked the patient's chart, his MAR, his identification bracelet, and any other places where this information is routinely listed. She could even have asked the patient whether he'd ever had any reaction to a medication.

But this incident has still another lesson for nurses: Don't let patients, family, friends—or even prison guards—interfere with your nursing actions. You're responsible for your actions, and you know how they should be carried out. Don't let a tense situation make you deviate from the correct procedure.

Failing to be cautious with the Add-Vantage system

A number of I.V. medications you commonly administer are now available in a drug-delivery system called Add-Vantage (manufactured by Abbott Laboratories). This system includes a vial of undiluted medication that screws into a special minibag of diluent (5% dextrose or normal saline solution).

Living up to its name, this system offers several advantages. For example, you can catch potential errors by double-checking the labels on the vial and minibag of diluent before reconstituting *and* before administering it. Also, it eliminates needles, syringes, and separate diluent vials. And it doesn't require refrigeration or special storage because the drug and diluent aren't mixed until administered.

But no system is perfect. Here are two problems that have cropped up with Add-Vantage:

• *Nurses have forgotten to remove the plug.* When the plug remains in the vial, patients receive only the diluent—a medication error or omission. You should manipulate the container to remove the stopper and mix the contents of the vial with the piggyback fluid. To do this, push the vial inward to "puff up" the bag, then grasp the vial's inner stopper through the bag walls and pull it out of the vial. Invert the vial and minibag together several times to mix the drug and diluent.

• *The system has malfunctioned.* Even when nurses have removed the plug, the attached rubber stopper has remained in place, preventing mixing. This can be corrected by manipulating the plug back into the vial's stopper and starting over. If the problem goes undetected, plain diluent will be administered.

To reinforce the mixing step, Abbott Laboratories now distributes a special sticker to fit across the hanger of the I.V. minibag. The label, which must be removed before the bag is hung, reminds you to "Pull stopper and mix drug before use."

You can make sure that the contents of the vial have been emptied into the I.V. minibag by looking through the vial's clear bottom just before hanging the container. (Do this in good light; we've heard of night-shift nurses who've mixed the drug diluent in darkened rooms, then found out in the morning that the vial didn't empty into the minibag.) If powder or fluid remains in the vial, or if the rubber stopper is still in place, something has gone wrong. Report malfunctions to your pharmacist. And remind him to inform Abbott Laboratories.

Error Number	**Not using three separate lines when transcribing an order that calls for two tablets**

185

A doctor ordered the sustaincd-release form of "morphine, MS Contin, 60 mg q12h." Because the pharmacy usually dispensed this drug in 30 mg tablets, the nurse transcribed the order in the medication administration record (MAR) like this:

MS Contin 60 mg
2 tabs PO q 12 h prn pain

Without notifying the nurses, the pharmacy dispensed 60 mg tablets, which had recently become available. So the nurses gave two of the 60 mg tablets with each dose. A discrepancy in the narcotics inventory sheet alerted them to the error.

With better communication between the two departments, this error never would have occurred. It also could have been prevented if the nurse had transcribed the order more clearly. You should use *three* separate lines in the MAR to transcribe orders when other than a single tablet or capsule is needed for a dose. Here's what to do.

On the first line, write the drug name and total dose ordered. The number of tablets or capsules, along with the strength of each, goes in parentheses on the second line. If you aren't sure about the strength, call the pharmacy. On the third line, complete the order by recording the administration route, frequency, and other information. Here's how the order for MS Contin should have been written:

MS Contin 60 mg
(2 × 30 mg)
PO q 12 h prn pain

Remember, the first line should always include the dose for single-ingredient drugs, not the number of tablets or capsules. For example, "K-Dur, 2 tablets" is unclear, because it comes in 10 mEq and 20 mEq tablets. Even if only one strength is available, you should include it when transcribing the order. Chances are, another strength will be marketed sooner or later. Your pharmacists should also follow this recommendation when labeling unit doses and when building a computerized drug inventory.

The nurse who transcribed this order did one thing right: She indicated that the nurses should give two tablets. When more than one tablet or capsule is needed per dose, someone is likely to forget and give only one. That's a good reason for pharmacists to dispense medications in the exact dose whenever possible. Also, they could consider formulating a capsule or supplying a liquid form when a patient must take a large number of tablets for one dose. Besides being more conevenient for the patient, it cuts down on the potential for making errors, because the nurse and patient have fewer tablets to handle.

Notes:

Error
Number

186

Confusing "Cardene" with "codeine"

A doctor ordered "Cardene, 30 mg P.O., q8h" for a patient who had a history of migraine headaches. Cardene is the trade name for nicardipine, a new calcium channel blocker similar to nifedipine (Procardia). The nurse misread this written order as "codeine." She got the dose from the unit's narcotics cabinet and gave it to her patient.

The next day, the doctor discovered the error on the patient's medication administration record. He told the nurse, who'd never heard of Cardene.

Pharmacists should alert nurses to new drugs and provide information to supplement any drug reference book on the unit. That hadn't happened at this hospital. So even if this nurse had wanted information about Cardene, she wouldn't have found anything about it in the drug book.

This patient had taken Cardene before, which she told the nurse later when questioned about her medications. That underscores the importance of getting a complete drug history as soon as possible after a patient is admitted.

Notes:

Being involved in same-name mix-ups

William Tompkins and Rebecca Tompkins, unrelated patients, were assigned to the same nursing unit. Both were receiving I.V. antibiotics for systemic infections. Rebecca had a history of penicillin sensitivity.

One evening, Rebecca's nurse took a piggyback of Timentin from the unit refrigerator. This antibiotic contains ticarcillin disodium and clavulanate potassium. It had been intended for William. Soon after the infusion began, Rebecca broke out in a rash on her arms and trunk. Her nurse stopped the infusion and administered an antihistamine as ordered.

The pharmacist who'd prepared the bag of Timentin had labeled it with the patient's last name and first initial only. And the nurse had just looked at the last name. In Rebecca's room, she thought she'd properly identified the patient, so she didn't realize her error.

Unfortunately, mix-ups like this aren't uncommon. The easiest solution is to put two unrelated patients with the same surname on different nursing units. If this is impossible, unit secretaries, pharmacists, and nurses who transcribe orders and dispense or administer medications should always use the patient's first and last names in all written and verbal references.

You could also consider the "name alert" fluorescent stickers sold by some companies. These can be placed strategically on charts, I.V. labels, and so on to make everyone aware that two patients on the same unit have the same last name.

Notes:

Error
Number

188

Confusing "AU" with "OU"

A doctor wrote the following order for an 8-year-old boy:

Colymycin drops iii ou tid

The attending nurse obtained the medication and administered the solution in each eye. Almost immediately the boy cried out in pain. The nurse was shocked and bewildered and ran to get another nurse on the unit. The other nurse quickly discovered what had happened when she saw the medication order. She knew the boy had recently developed an inner ear infection—something the administering nurse didn't know because she was new to the unit. She misinterpreted the abbreviation AU (each ear) for OU (each eye).

They called the boy's doctor who gave a telephone order for eye irrigation. The boy suffered no further ill effects in his eyes and the Colymycin was properly administered in each ear.

The best way to prevent such an error is to not use these abbreviations. But if you see it, always question the order.

Notes:

_____

_____

_____

_____

_____

Mistaking the term "midnight" and the abbreviations used for 12 noon and 12 midnight

Error Number

189

A doctor wrote the following order:

(handwritten order) Decadron 4 mg IV q 6 h until midnight 1/30/90

The nurse interpreting the order assumed midnight to be between 1/30 and 1/31. So she continued to give the medication during the day on January 30th. The attending doctor questioned the nurse as to why his patient was still receiving medication when he specified the time for termination. The nurse explained her interpretation of the order. The doctor realized what had happened and explained he intended the medication to be stopped midnight between 1/29 and 1/30.

According to the Time Service Division of the Naval Observatory in Washington, D.C., this is a common problem. They recommend the following solutions.

1. Designate midnight using the date falling before and after midnight. For example, 12 midnight on 1/30 should be listed as 12 midnight (1/29–1/30).

2. Use schedules (have doctors' orders) that specify 12:01 or 11:59 (this seems impractical for hospitals). This system is used by railroads.

3. Use military time systems. 0100 (1 AM) to 0000 (12 midnight). This system is in use by airlines and the military. Unfortunately, most people (including military personnel) believe that 2400 is the last number in the system but there's no such number—it's 0000 or 0 h. Using 2400 makes one think it is the end of the day, which it is not.

Another issue which is confusing is whether midnight is 12 a.m. and noon is 12 p.m. (right) or vice versa (wrong). Again, different people have different opinions. This can also lead to medication error. The National Bureau of Standards recommends that, because of their ambiguity, the abbreviations 12 a.m. and 12 p.m. never be used. They suggest the terms noon and midnight be used instead or, more precisely, 12 noon and 12 midnight with no abbreviation.

Misinterpreting a poorly written doctor's order

A 70-year-old woman, an insulin-controlled diabetic patient, was receiving 80 mg of prednisone daily. This dosage had been administered for two weeks. The patient's doctor wanted to begin withdrawal of the steroid and wrote an order to "decrease prednisone 5 mg daily."

A unit clerk transcribed the order and the new dose listed was 5 mg daily—not 75 mg daily. This was checked by a nurse who evidently interpreted the order in the same way. The following day the patient received only 5 mg (her insulin dosage remained the same).

Later that day, the patient collapsed and the hospital resuscitation team was called. Administration of glucose assisted in reviving her. Blood glucose at the time of collapse was less than 50 mg per ml.

The situation could have been prevented by a more clearly phrased doctor's order. What should have been written was "Decrease prednisone by 5 mg daily," or better yet, "Decrease prednisone to 75 mg daily." Nursing personnel must also be aware of the need for gradual withdrawal from corticosteroids when patients receive such high doses for more than a week.

Notes:

Using an obsolete abbreviation

A nurse's medication card read:

T pramnic syrup 3 T po qid.

A student nurse interpreted this dosage to be 3T or 3 table-spoonsful. Instead of 5 ml, a pediatric patient received 45 ml of the medication. Aside from extreme drowsiness, the child had no other ill effects. He was observed for 24 hours. The student nurse had questioned her instructor and a team leader; yet she was told to go ahead and give the dose.

Obvious advice is to insist upon proper terms and symbols. There is no longer any use for the apothecary system and its abbreviations. The metric system has taken over in medicine.

Although these apothecary abbreviations are not to be used, unfortunately, they are still found sometimes in doctors' orders and are transcribed onto medication records. We should campaign against their use—obviously for good reason.

Some people were taught that capital "T" meant tablespoonful and small "t" meant teaspoonful. These abbreviations are also used in cooking. The doctor's apothecary abbreviation for the number one looked like a capital T. The sign for dram looked like a 3.

Notes:

_____

_____

_____

_____

Error
Number

192

Not knowing about treatment of acetaminophen overdose

A patient with an acetaminophen overdose was admitted to an emergency department and therapy began with the antidote, acetylcysteine. She was then transferred to a special care unit where therapy was continued. The doctor's original order read:

Mucomyst 20% 3.5 g PO q 4 h

Because the nurse was familiar with the use of Mucomyst as a mucolytic, she questioned the oral use of the drug and the dose. She tried unsuccessfully to get further information on this from her supervisor, two other nurses, and a doctor. The package insert mentioned only its mucolytic activity. Finally, after considerable delay, she changed the 3.5 g to 3.5 ml (3.5 g would be 17.5 ml) and administered it orally.

The incident occurred on a Sunday night. On Monday morning, pharmacy dispensed the balance of the order, properly labeled as 3.5 g = 17.5 ml. However, four days later, a pharmacist noted that the majority of the Mucomyst dispensed was being returned. After floor personnel were questioned, the original error was discovered and it was determined that the patient had not received the proper dose at any time during the four-day period. Fortunately, the patient survived the error. The error could have been prevented if one of the nurses had contacted the pharmacist on call or if a pharmacist had been on duty at the time the drug was ordered.

Notes:

_____

_____

_____

_____

Giving an overdose of estrogen to a patient

Premarin 0.625 mg was ordered for a patient. No 0.625 mg tablets were available in the pharmacy. The pharmacy technician decided that he would give an equal dose by using a number of tablets of a "lesser" strength. Apparently he thought the dose was 6.25 mg. He placed five 1.25 mg Premarin tablets together in a unit-dose package and placed these in the patient's bin of a unit-dose cart. The medication nurse, upon receiving the cart, returned with the dose to question the use of the five tablets, and was told by the technician that the dose was correct. The pharmacist was not consulted about the dose by the technician or the nurse, although he was present in the pharmacy at the time. The patient, who had gynecologic problems in the past, received the dose and exhibited vaginal bleeding three days later. The cause of the bleeding was later discovered and explained to the patient.

Two important points need to be made in considering this medication error. First, pharmacists must make every effort not to substitute smaller dose tablets or capsules to equal a larger dose. Not only do patients have more tablets to swallow, there's a greater chance an error will occur or that only part of the dose will be given.

Second, if you do find yourself needing to give more than one or two capsules, vials, tablets, ampules, etc., chances are there's something wrong. So check with another nurse or your pharmacist.

Notes:

_____

_____

_____

_____

_____

Error
Number

194

Not knowing the difference between enteral and parenteral alimentation

A 60-year-old man, unconscious as a result of a cardiopulmonary arrest with resuscitation, was receiving enteral alimentation, through a Silastic nasogastric (NG) tube. The 24-hour supply of 3,000 ml of nutrient (Vivonex) was being divided into three bottles daily, each administered over eight hours by infusion pump. Powdered nutrient was dissolved in sterile water for irrigation contained in liter bottles with screw caps. The screw cap was modified to accept an I.V. solution administration set with a pump chamber and the Luer-Lok tip of the set connected directly to the NG tube. The solution set and screw cap were to be changed every 24 hours.

On the second day, the person placing the fresh set and cap on the first bottle that day connected the line to a central venous catheter instead of to the NG tube. The patient received approximately 400 ml of solution before the error was recognized.

Although the patient experienced seizures, it could not be determined with certainty whether these were due to inadvertent I.V. infusion or to the patient's previous cerebral anoxia. The patient was placed on prophylactic antibiotic therapy. He experienced no fevers after the incident. Since the patient was also already on a ventilator, respiratory difficulty, if it occurred, was not readily recognizable.

Obviously, the person who connected the solution to the I.V. catheter did not think about what he or she was doing. The container was not an I.V. bottle; it had a special screw cap. The solution was not a clear liquid. The individual should have been aware of what type of therapy the patient was receiving and of the difference between enteral and parenteral alimentation (some are confused by the term "hyperalimentation" and do not differentiate).

There are other considerations. A pharmacist prepared the final solutions and labeled the bottles with labels normally used for I.V. therapy. If enteral alimentation is to be used, off-color labels should be utilized. They should prominently warn that the solution is "for enteral use—not for injection." These labels would help greatly to prevent errors in administration.

Tubing used with enteral alimentation should have connections that cannot fit I.V. catheters. Some companies manufacture infusion pump sets for use specifically with enteral alimentation. The tubing will not accommodate an I.V. catheter. Other companies should make such sets available from some manufacturers of enteral alimentation products, but these are not easily used with infusion pumps.

Lastly, if enteral and parenteral alimentation are being used in your institution, make sure that hospital personnel receive the educational support necessary to understand and utilize this type of therapy properly.

Notes:

_____

_____

_____

_____

_____

Failing to use a manufacturer's package properly

An order was received in the pharmacy for birth control tablets to be given four times daily. The patient for whom the order was written had vaginal bleeding. Seven brown tablets remained out of a package originally containing 28 tablets. These were dispensed and administered for the first seven doses.

After two days, a fresh package of birth control pills was opened. The person administering medications was surprised to see a color difference in the tablets dispensed by the pharmacy the second time. The second tablets were pink; this was questioned. It was discovered that the original seven tablets dispensed that were brown in color were actually inert tablets. These remained in the package after the active pills (pink) had been punched out. Someone had returned the remaining inert tablet portion of the blister to stock. The patient was still bleeding after the seven inert doses.

The person using the active tablets should have made certain that the remaining tablets were discarded. Preferably, the iron tablets should have been punched out as soon as the package was opened for use other than as birth control pills.

Notes:

_____

_____

_____

_____

_____

Not using the correct route of administration for kanamycin prophylaxis

A 91-year-old woman was to undergo bowel resection. A surgeon wrote the following order as part of preoperative bowel preparation:

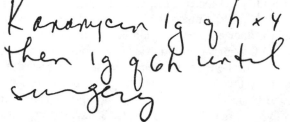

No route of adminstration was specified. The first dose was requested verbally from the pharmacy as "Kantrex 500 mg I.M." Subsequent doses were scheduled in the nursing medication administration records to be given intramuscularly. When the pharmacist received the written order and saw the dosage ordered, it was obvious to him that the drug was meant to be given orally.

This error could have had serious consequences. The nephrotoxicity and ototoxicity of systemic kanamycin is well known. If the drug were given systemically in the dosage ordered, these side effects would be likely to occur. Because the oral dosage form (capsule) is not appreciably absorbed, this form is used in doses much higher than those used systemically. Its local effect within the bowel lumen reduces bowel flora before operation.

One of the factors that led to this error was that no route of administration was specified by the doctor. Because not everyone is familiar with the oral dosage form, and because the use of kanamycin by parenteral route or as an irrigation is better known, the lack of specification of route of administration led to the belief that the intramuscular (I.M.) route was to be used.

Personnel responsible for scheduling and administering medications in this hospital showed a lack of information about the dosage range of kanamycin and about the serious side effects of the drug that are more likely with high doses. If this had been known, the error would not have occurred. Hospitals must have policies that require pharmacists to see a written order before any nonemergency drug is dispensed.

Error
Number

197

Failing to use the correct dropper to administer a dose of liquid tranquilizer

An inpatient prescription written for fluphenazine hydrochloride (Prolixin Elixir) was filled in the pharmacy in a 4 oz. pharmacy glass bottle. It was labeled as 0.5 mg/ml. Since the dose prescribed was 5 mg, the pharmacist who filled the prescription assumed that a floor employee would use a dose measurer to pour 10 ml of the 0.5 mg/ml liquid. However, someone, apparently thinking it would be more convenient to use a dose-graded dropper to measure the dose, placed a dropper from an empty bottle of Stelazine Concentrate into the Prolixin bottle. The dropper cap fit perfectly. The measurements on the Stelazine Concentrate (10 mg/ml) dropper are 10 mg, 8 mg, and 5 mg. Each of several doses of 5 mg was measured by using the 5 mg increment on the Stelazine dropper. The dose actually administered then was 0.25 mg of Prolixin, a good deal less than the 5 mg intended.

Several factors contributed to this medication error. First and obvious is that droppers meant for one particular medication are not interchangeable for use with another. They should not be used to cap a bottle of another drug, even on a temporary basis, such as if the original nondropper cap was lost or broken. The dropper itself in this case clearly stated "Stelazine." If this had been read, perhaps the error would not have occurred.

The labeling placed on the bottle in the pharmacy is also open to criticism. The label should have stated the volume of elixir necessary to administer the 5 mg dose. If prepackaged unit doses of liquids were utilized, this type of error would not have been possible.

Notes: _____

_____

_____

_____

_____

Using coined names

Several years ago, a relatively inexperienced evening pharmacist received an order for "Black and White, 30 ml hs prn." The only black and white the pharmacist knew of was Scotch whisky. The whisky had been stored by the pharmacy for some time and was dispensed occasionally by doctor's order. This is what was dispensed. No complaint was voiced by the patient. The doctor who wrote the order claimed that "everybody knows that Black and White is a laxative mixture containing the equivalent of 5 ml of aromatic cascara fluid extract and 30 ml of milk of magnesia." Everyone, of course, except people who've never heard of a black and white! It is easy to understand how coined names and abbreviations evolve.

Obviously, everyone does not know what these unique "nicknames" mean, thus errors occur. Health professionals waste time clarifying orders and therapy is delayed as a result. Community pharmacists are particularly vulnerable when they receive prescriptions for coined-name drugs that are familiar to only those who work within the institution where the doctor practices. For example, a dermatologist routinely prescribed "T.M.C.," an abbreviation for triamcinolone. Several calls from community practitioners were made asking what this was.

In another example, when a topical solution mixture of three antibiotics was being used in hip surgery, a lazy doctor ordered "chicken soup" rather than spelling out the lengthy formula. Nurses and pharmacists knew what the orthopedist wanted. But can you envision this medical record being used in a court case, or even worse, chicken soup being used? Other such orders have included "pink lady" (tincture of belladonna, Maalox, and phenobarbital elixir) or "dynamite" (Dulcolax).

Most Pharmacy and Therapeutics Committees have rules on the books stating that no chemical symbols be used in writing orders and that there be an approved list of abbreviations (this is a JCAHO requirement). When a complex formula is consistently prescribed, a descriptive name for this product should be approved by the Pharmacy and Therapeutics Committee for use only within the institution. The name and exact formula must appear in the formulary and on container labels. Every effort must be made to resist creating unofficial names.

214

Error
Number

199

Writing a patient's name and bed number directly on labels of unit-dose products

After a unit-dose cart supply was checked and delivered to the patient care area by a pharmacist, he received a new order for ampicillin 500 mg P.O. q6h. The pharmacist took three doses, enough to last until the next cart fill, and placed them in a Ziploc bag. He wrote the name of the patient and bed number on the bag and sent it to the nursing unit for the nurse to place in the patient's drug bin on the cart. The pharmacist did not notice that, earlier in the day, someone else had dispensed those very capsules and had written a name and bed number directly on the label of one of them. When the medication was later discontinued, the capsules were returned to stock but the name and bed number were not crossed off.

Upon receipt, a nurse removed one dose from the bag, then administered it to the wrong patient—the same patient for whom it had already been ordered and discontinued. Later, when the nurse saw the name and bed number written on the Ziploc bag, she discovered that an error had been made. She wrongly assumed that the name and the bed number written on the unit-dose package label identified the patient for whom it was intended (she remembered seeing an earlier order for that patient, but was unaware it had been discontinued). Of course, if the nurse had followed procedure by checking the patient's medication administration record, the error would not have occurred, but the name and bed number on the label contributed to the error. There is a danger that similar errors could occur with stat doses and other miscellaneous, one-time-only items, as well as with drugs dispensed to update unit-dose carts before the next fill.

One of the major cost-saving advantages of unit-dose packaging is that dispensed but unadministered medications may be returned to stock for reissue without fear of loss of identity or hygienic conditions. But writing the patient name and bed number directly on the label of nonroutinely dispensed doses may later lead to error if the dose is returned. This practice should be discouraged. A supplemental label that can be torn off if the drug is returned would be more acceptable. Alternatively, all doses delivered after normal cart fill should go directly into patient bins or should be placed in Ziploc bags, which are then labeled. If returned, the doses may be removed and returned to stock.

Giving an overdose of vinblastine because the written order was misinterpreted

A cancer patient was scheduled to receive 3 mg of vinblastine daily for 5 days but instead received a seven-fold overdose of vinblastine, resulting in death. How could this happen?

To have syringes of vinblastine for Autosyringe available when the patient was ready to pick them up, a nurse working with the patient's doctor would call the outpatient oncology nurse with the order. The outpatient nurse would record the order on the patient's clinic chart and phone the satellite pharmacist to have him prepare the order she just transcribed. The pharmacist would prepare the doses and have them ready in a "will call" area. When the patient arrived with the actual prescription, the pharmacist would check it against what was made and then dispense the drug.

The outpatient nurse phoned the pharmacist for five vinblastine 20 mg syringes. She said one was to be infused I.V. daily for 5 days. The pharmacist prepared the syringes and placed them in the "will call" area. When the patient arrived, the outpatient nurse took the medication from the "will call" area and gave it to the patient without giving the prescription to the pharmacist. The prescription was actually written for 3 mg daily for 5 days. The nurse never checked nor did the pharmacist. After 3 days of therapy the patient became ill and the error was discovered. The patient eventually died.

The error occurred either with the office nurse's verbal transmission or with the outpatient nurse's call to the pharmacist. It was never determined for sure.

Drugs with as much potential for toxicity as anticancer drugs should never be dispensed secondary to a verbal order. If necessary, the order transmission process can be hastened with the use of fax machines. Written orders must be interpreted by both nurses and pharmacists.

INDEX